MEDICAL PROCEDURES, TESTING AND TECHNOLOGY

ULTRASOUND IN BONE FRACTURES

FROM ASSESSMENT TO THERAPY

MEDICAL PROCEDURES, TESTING AND TECHNOLOGY

Additional books in this series can be found on Nova's website under the Series tab.

Additional e-books in this series can be found on Nova's website under the e-book tab.

BIOMEDICAL DEVICES AND THEIR APPLICATIONS

Additional books in this series can be found on Nova's website under the Series tab.

Additional e-books in this series can be found on Nova's website under the e-book tab.

MEDICAL PROCEDURES, TESTING AND TECHNOLOGY

ULTRASOUND IN BONE FRACTURES

FROM ASSESSMENT TO THERAPY

CHRISTIANO B. MACHADO, PH.D.

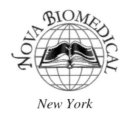

New York

Copyright © 2013 by Nova Science Publishers, Inc.

All rights reserved. No part of this book may be reproduced, stored in a retrieval system or transmitted in any form or by any means: electronic, electrostatic, magnetic, tape, mechanical photocopying, recording or otherwise without the written permission of the Publisher.

For permission to use material from this book please contact us:
Telephone 631-231-7269; Fax 631-231-8175
Web Site: http://www.novapublishers.com

NOTICE TO THE READER

The Publisher has taken reasonable care in the preparation of this book, but makes no expressed or implied warranty of any kind and assumes no responsibility for any errors or omissions. No liability is assumed for incidental or consequential damages in connection with or arising out of information contained in this book. The Publisher shall not be liable for any special, consequential, or exemplary damages resulting, in whole or in part, from the readers' use of, or reliance upon, this material. Any parts of this book based on government reports are so indicated and copyright is claimed for those parts to the extent applicable to compilations of such works.

Independent verification should be sought for any data, advice or recommendations contained in this book. In addition, no responsibility is assumed by the publisher for any injury and/or damage to persons or property arising from any methods, products, instructions, ideas or otherwise contained in this publication.

This publication is designed to provide accurate and authoritative information with regard to the subject matter covered herein. It is sold with the clear understanding that the Publisher is not engaged in rendering legal or any other professional services. If legal or any other expert assistance is required, the services of a competent person should be sought. FROM A DECLARATION OF PARTICIPANTS JOINTLY ADOPTED BY A COMMITTEE OF THE AMERICAN BAR ASSOCIATION AND A COMMITTEE OF PUBLISHERS.

Additional color graphics may be available in the e-book version of this book.

Library of Congress Cataloging-in-Publication Data

ISBN: 978-1-62808-506-8

Library of Congress Control Number: 2013945714

Published by Nova Science Publishers, Inc. † New York

To my beloved wife Daniela, with all my love and affection ... you are my support on this Earth! Thank you for everything!

Contents

Foreword	Wagner C. A. Pereira and Pascal Laugier	ix
Preface		xiii
Acknowledgments		xv
Section I	**Bone Tissue**	1
Chapter 1	Bone Tissue Histology and Biology	3
Chapter 2	Bone Tissue Mechanics	19
Chapter 3	The Fracture Healing Phenomenon	37
Section II	**Basics of Ultrasound Physics**	53
Chapter 4	Acoustic Wave Propagation	55
Chapter 5	The Piezoelectric Effect and Acoustic Transducers	75
Chapter 6	The Scattering of Ultrasound Waves and Ultrasound Imaging	89
Chapter 7	Ultrasound Propagation in Bones	113
Section III	**Ultrasound as a Clinical Assessment Tool for Fracture Healing**	143
Chapter 8	Ultrasound Imaging and Bone Fractures	145
Chapter 9	Quantitative Ultrasound Techniques and Bone Fractures	167

Section IV	**Ultrasound as a Therapeutic Tool for Fracture Healing**	**203**
Chapter 10	Bioeffects of Ultrasound in Fracture Regeneration	**205**
Chapter 11	Therapeutic Ultrasound in Fractures: State of the Art	**215**
Index		**251**

Foreword

It is a real pleasure to be invited to give a foreword on this book from Dr. Christiano Machado. About 10 years ago he decided to enter in the biomedical engineering field and applied for the Master in Science course in Brazil, finishing with a successful production after two years. Dr. Machado continued his studies by applying for a joint supervision regime doctorate ("Cotutelle program") between Brazil and France where he developed most of his skills in ultrasound applied to bone. Now he gives an important step in his career by transforming his experience into a book that, we are sure, will be an important state-of-the-art text to those interested in entering the field. Ultrasound has been traditionally applied in soft tissues and only recently a stronger scientific effort has been gathered toward bone characterization and potential therapeutic effects. It is still an open research subject but a lot of important issues have been addressed and important results achieved. We want to say that we are proud to participate in the first stages of Dr. Machado´s carreer, and since he is young there is much more to come.

As that of many other scientific fields, the history of ultrasound clinical use for bone is made of booms and regressions. Clinical bone imaging technology is largely based on using X-rays. But since X-rays imaging does not provide all of the information that is needed by clinicians, particularly for bone strength assessment, in the second part of the twentieth century researchers turned to ultrasound. The first investigations using ultrasound for bone assessment reported in the late 1950s were designed to monitor fracture healing. Despite the publication of interesting results, it took 25 years before diagnostic ultrasound succeeded in attracting clinicians in a completely different field, that of osteoporotic fracture risk prediction.

In parallel and approximately in the same period, efforts have been made to enhance fracture healing using physical methods, including ultrasound stimulation among others, a method which was known as low-intensity pulsed ultrasound (LIPUS). The first clinical report that ultrasound stimulates fracture healing traces back to early 1950s, but only in the 1980s we observed the attention of basic scientists and physicians. Since then, a growing body of evidence was provided on the potential of LIPUS to enhance fracture healing by scientific studies, from *in vitro* and animal studies to clinical trials and case series. Interestingly, one of the first (if not the first one) patent filled on LIPUS technology, in 1982, was authored by a Brazilian researcher, Luis R. Duarte, from the University of São Paulo, Brazil.

The late 1990s and early 2000s have been the golden age of quantitative ultrasound methods to assess bone, a field commonly referred to as Bone QUS. Those years, engineers, scientists and clinicians combined their efforts; many ultrasound technologies were invented and made available to benefit the patients in order to improve the prediction of fracture risk and the therapeutic management. However, diagnostic QUS-based methods have failed to emerge as an alternative to X-ray. The LIPUS technology has been made commercially available to clinicians in those years, but is still not widely clinically used.

Despite the fact that ultrasound is used clinically, both for diagnosis and therapy, the interaction of ultrasound waves with bone is by no means well understood, hampered by the structural complexity of bone. This probably partly explains the current absence of widespread clinical use of ultrasound for bone diagnosis and therapy. It is for this reason that ultrasonic propagation in bone has been under intensive investigation during the last decade, with a particular emphasis on modeling.

Modeling can be seen as a major need in order: (1) to relate QUS variables to relevant bone biomechanical properties and to quantify these properties; (2) to gain deeper insight into mechanisms by which therapeutic effects on bone are mediated; (3) to integrate multiscale knowledge; and finally (4) to optimize QUS measurements and LIPUS protocols and to drive future experiments. The field is vivid and continuously stimulates productive research.

In this book, Dr. Christiano Machado provides the reader with a timely and brilliant compilation of the most important and most recent accomplishments that have been made in the field of ultrasound in bone fractures. The book is intended to give an overview of the field and consists of chapters detailing theoretical and experimental aspects of the interaction phenomenon between ultrasound waves and bone. It has been written in accessible language to both engineers and health workers. We have no doubt that it will serve as a handy reference for the workers on the field and will be able to provide a clear perspective for readers who are interested in learning more about this domain. In closing, we would like to thank Dr. Christiano Machado who has undertaken this invaluable work to the benefit of the whole community by sharing his deep knowledge of the field.

Dr. Wagner C. A. Pereira
Ultrasound Laboratory - Biomedical Engineering Program –
COPPE/Federal University of Rio de Janeiro - Brazil

Dr. Pascal Laugier
Laboratoire d'Imagerie Paramétrique – University Paris-Sorbonne 6 –
France

Preface

My first contact with science was in 1999, when I began my scientific initiation at the Physical Therapy Department, Estácio de Sá University, in the city of Nova Friburgo, state of Rio de Janeiro, Brazil. Although I had developed some works in Exercise Physiology at that time, ultrasound appeared in my life in 2001, during a course of electro-thermo-sonotherapy, in which we learned how to use equipment like ultrasound, electrical stimulation, infrared and short waves therapy in a clinical practice. Since that period I was always wondering: how the author of a book "A" or "B" can say that ultrasound is efficient for pain relief, inflammation, muscle relaxation etc., without scientific evidence in the human body; or how physical therapists can continue to use therapeutic approaches relying on empirical hypotheses?

From 2003 to 2005, during my Masters in Biomedical Engineering at the Federal University of Rio de Janeiro, with Dr. Wagner Pereira, I finally went deeper in the acoustical sciences, developing a study about the use of ultrasound backscattering signals to characterize *in vitro* healthy and pathological hepatic tissues. For a health science professional, it was not an easy task to think like an engineer or a physicist. However, it was necessary to follow course lectures on mathematics, computational sciences, signal processing and statistics. Therefore, I have become a "two-dimensional researcher" (Health and Exact Sciences). I had the opportunity to continue my collaboration with Dr. Pereira, together with Dr. Pascal Laugier from the *Laboratoire d'Imagerie Paramétrique* (University of Paris 6, France), during my PhD (2007 – 2011), however focusing my research on the use of quantitative ultrasound in fracture healing monitoring. This book was conceived out of this experience.

Ultrasound has a twofold perspective for bone fracture healing: therapy and diagnosis/follow-up. Literature has shown that low-intensity pulsed ultrasound stimulation (LIPUS) can enhance fracture healing, although the mechanisms underlying this stimulation are not completely understood. At the same time, ultrasonic waves have been applied for medical imaging techniques, as well as for the use of quantitative ultrasound (QUS) in an attempt to assess callus tissue status. Nonetheless, for this last approach, research is still at the initial stages. Indeed some papers have been published, but a lot is still to come, until clinicians accept QUS techniques in their clinical practice.

This book aims at presenting these two applications of ultrasound in bone fractures. First of all, bone tissue is presented in the first three chapters. We will discuss bone biology, biomechanics and the fracture healing process, always focusing on important aspects for the later chapters. From chapter 4 to 7, ultrasound will be explored: the acoustic wave propagation and basic equations, the piezoelectric effect and beamforming, the scattering of ultrasound, imaging techniques, and the propagation of ultrasound in bones. Chapters 8 and 9 will deal with ultrasound as an assessment tool for fractures (from imaging to QUS), and finally chapters 10 and 11 will explain how ultrasound can accelerate the fracture healing process, always presenting the most relevant scientific evidence in these fields.

I hope this book can be very helpful for students, who are initiating this research domain, as well as for seniors, to get updated about recent findings. Since I am not a physicist or an engineer, but a PhD in Physical Sciences, my intention here is to present the subject from a clinical perspective, but never letting aside the mathematical and physical basis of the ultrasound interaction with bone and fractures.

Christiano B. Machado
PhD in Acoustical Physics - University of Paris VI - France
PhD in Biomedical Engineering –
Federal University of Rio de Janeiro - Brazil
Director of the Biomedical Ultrasound Laboratory –
Estácio de Sá University - Rio de Janeiro - Brazil

Acknowledgments

This book would not have been possible without the support of many people. I would like to express my gratitude to my PhD supervisors, Dr. Wagner Pereira and Dr. Pascal Laugier, who were very helpful and always offered invaluable support and guidance.

My deepest gratitude is due to people who gave me important help during my PhD thesis: doctors Frédéric Padilla, Maryline Talmant, Julien Grondin, and Mathilde Granke. Thanks to doctors Kay Raum and Daniel Rohrbach from the Julius Wolff Institut (Berlin) for helpful discussions about ultrasound and fracture healing.

Thanks a lot to my good friends Bill and Aïda Hamilton for English editing.

Special thanks also to Estácio de Sá University, in Rio de Janeiro, the Institution where I have become a physical therapist, and where I conduct nowadays my research in biomedical ultrasound. Thanks to Prof. Carlos Eduardo Neves and Edil Luis Santos for presenting me to the wonderful world of science. Thanks to all my colleagues and lovely students from the Physical Therapy Department.

Not forgetting my dear friends from Paris, Dorothée, Sylvain, Thien-Ly, Jacques, Guillaume, Jean-Gabriel and Herga, Quentin, Sara, Josquin, Emmanuel and Michelle Fleck, Mahmoud, and Giácomo.

I would also like to convey thanks to the Brazilian Ministry of Science and Technology, the agencies CAPES and FAPERJ for providing the financial means and laboratory facilities for my research.

I wish to express my love and gratitude to my beloved family (Daniela, Aida, Joaquim, Fabrício, Joaquim Jr., Élida) for their understanding and endless love.

To God my Father, I am (and I will always be) thankful for His strength which has upheld me for years and years, mainly during 2009, when I lived alone in Paris. I would be nothing without Your holy presence.

Section I - Bone Tissue

Chapter 1

Bone Tissue Histology and Biology

Abstract

From both micro and macroscopic point of view, bone tissue is a complex living structure, presenting several functions in the human body: support, protection, biomechanical levers, and ions reservoir. Two important mechanical characteristics of the bone are stiffness and flexibility. The mechanics of this tissue depends on bone biology, and four types of cells are responsible to assure its functions: osteoblasts (for mineralization regulation), osteoclasts (for bone resorption), osteocytes (mature osteoblasts) and bone lining cells. According to its porosity, bone can be classified in trabecular (highly porous, with non-calcified regions filled with marrow) and compact (low porosity, high density) bone. Bone growth is dependent on two basic phenomena: the intramembranous (or direct) and the endochondral (or indirect) ossification. In intramembranous ossification, mesenchymal cells transform directly into osteoblasts. In endochondral ossification, cartilage is produced from the recruitment, proliferation and differentiation of embryonic mesenchymal cells, then progressively mineralized and replaced by bony matrix. At initial stages of development, long bones have a region called epiphyseal plate, formed by hyaline cartilage, which is progressively substituted by ossified tissue.

1.1. Introduction

Bone tissue is the main component of the skeleton, and it presents several important functions in the human body: support for soft tissues and muscle activity; protection for vital organs and marrow; biomechanical levers; calcium, phosphate and other ions reservoir. In addition, it can act in the mechanical aspect of hearing and blood production (the bone marrow produces blood cells through hematopoiesis). It is considered a complex structure because of its complex properties, being divided for convenience into five different levels (Figure 1.1) according to Rho *et al*.: (1) a macrostructure: the cortical and cancellous bone; (2) a microstructure (from 10 to 500 μm), composed by the so called Haversian systems, osteons and trabeculae; (3) a sub-microstructure (de 1 a 10 μm): the lamellae; (4) a nanostructure (from 100 nm to 1 μm), composed by collagen fibers and minerals; and finally (5) a sub-nanostructure (less than 100 nm), which is represented by the molecular structure of the bone elements like minerals, collagen and other organic proteins.

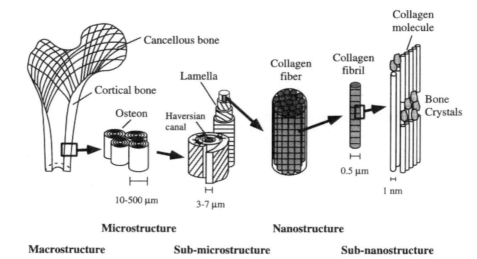

Figure 1.1. Hierarchical structural organization of bone tissue (Reprinted from Medical Engineering & Physics, vol. 20, n. 2, Jae-Young Rho, Liisa Kuhn-Spearing, Peter Zioupos, Mechanical properties and the hierarchical structure of bone, p. 93, Copyright (1998) with permission from Elsevier).

Stiffness and flexibility are two important mechanical features: the former comes from the presence of calcium phosphate (calcium hydroxyapatite) in the intercellular matrix; the latter originates from numerous embedded collagenous fibers within the matrix.

Bone mechanics depends intrinsically on bone biology. Four types of cells work metabolically to guarantee bone functions: osteoblasts (mineralization regulator of bone matrix), osteoclasts (responsible for bone resorption), osteocytes (mature osteoblasts responsible for tissue maintenance) and bone lining cells (little is known about their function).

Bones can be anatomically classified into five categories: the **long bones**, presenting a shaft (diaphysis) and forming most bones of the upper and lower limbs; the cube-shaped **short bones** mainly composed by trabecular bone and represented by the bones of the wrist and ankle; the **flat bones**, like bones in skull and sternum, with trabecular bone surrounded by two parallel layers of compact bone; the **irregular bones**, with irregular shapes (cannot be classified in another category), like the vertebrae and coxal bone; and finally the **sesamoid bones**, for example, the patella, which is a bone embedded in muscle tendons.

All the existing information about bones have only been gathered in the last decades. Bone is a difficult tissue to study because it is mineralized. Martin *et al.* (2010) explained that before the 1960s skeletal research was focused primarily on bone chemistry due to the great importance of mineral metabolism in physiology and medicine.

In this chapter, the basics of bone histology and biology will be presented.

1.2. Bone Cells and the Composition of Bone

Bone is composed of several biomolecules, including collagen, water, hydroxyapatite crystals, proteoglycans (decorin and biglycan, for example) and noncollagenous proteins (osteocalcin and osteopontin, for example). The basis of the mineral part of bone consists of hydroxyapatite crystals, with the molecular formula $Ca_{10}(PO_4)_6(OH)_2$. The role of proteoglycans and noncollagenous proteins is still unclear, but they may be responsible for the rate of mineralization or even acting like a chemoattractant for bone cells (Marks & Odgren, 2002).

The bone cells are represented by four specialized types of cells: osteoblasts, osteocytes, osteoclasts and the bone lining cells (Carter & Beaupré, 2001).

1.2.1. Osteoblasts

Osteoblasts are responsible for bone matrix production. They are fully differentiated mononuclear, cuboidal cells which produce the organic part of bone, called the osteoid (95% of type I collagen and 5% of noncollagenous proteins) from a Golgi apparatus and a endoplasmic reticulum. They are always side by side following an epithelial-like arrangement (Figure 1.2).

The mesenchymal cells originate osteoblasts through a differentiation process, and it appears to be initiated by mechanical stress. The apposition rate is the rate in which osteoblasts lay down osteoid (approximately 1 μm/day). Although the underlying mechanisms are not fully understood, these cells seem to regulate mineralization of bone matrix. It is possible to identify a boundary between the organic and calcified part of bone, the calcification (or mineralization) front.

1.2.2. Osteocytes

An **osteocyte** is a mature osteoblast. It is a flattened cell, exhibiting Golgi apparatus, endoplasmic reticulum and a nucleus with condensed chromatin. This type of cell is responsible for the maintenance of bone tissue, performing matrix synthesis and resorption to a limited extent. It can be found in spaces within the matrix called lacunae. Each lacuna incorporates only one osteocyte. The canaliculi are tunnels that make the communication among osteocytes (Figure 1.2).

An interesting finding is that an osteocyte may present cellular organelles characteristic of osteoblasts, functioning like an osteoblast, and on the other hand it may have lysosomal vacuoles and other features typical of phagocytic cells, acting like an osteoclast.

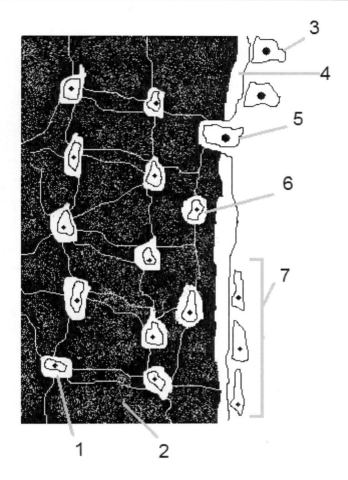

Figure 1.2. An illustration showing bone cells in action. It is possible to identify the osteocytes inside the lacunae (1) in the mineralized bone tissue (2). Osteoblasts originated from osteoprogenitor cells (3) lay down osteoid (4) to the formation of new osteocytes (5). Bone lining cells can be visualized in (6) localized in bone surface.

1.2.3. Osteoclasts

Osteoclasts are large, mobile and multinucleated cells, formed by fusion of monocytes from bone marrow (nonmineralized spaces within a bone). They are responsible for bone resorption through a sequence of chemical reactions. First of all, they erode bone by demineralizing the adjacent bone, and then utilize its enzymes to dissolve collagen (Figure 1.3).

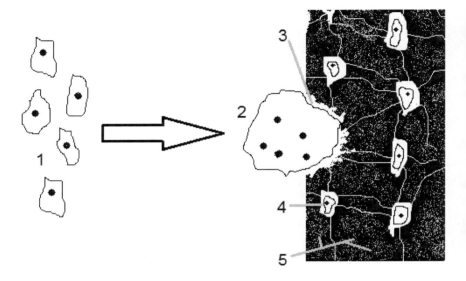

Figure 1.3. An illustration showing osteoclasts in action. A fusion of monocytes (1) originates the osteoclast, a multinuclear cell (2). The osteoclasts is responsible for bone resorption through a demineralization process (3). Osteocytes inside the lacunae (4) and bone mineralized matrix (5) can be also identified.

During resorption, osteoclasts rest on the bone surface. They show two plasma membrane specializations: a ruffled border (an infolded area for bone resorption) and a clear zone (with many actin microfilaments and no organelle surrounding the ruffled border, acting as an adhesion point between the osteoclast and bone matrix, and then creating a closed environment for resorption).

Osteoclast activity is coordinated by signaling molecules called cytokines, and by hormones (calcitonin and parathormone). They contain several Golgi apparatus, a high density of mitochondria and a great amount of lysosomal vesicles (Majeska, 2009).

1.2.4. Bone Lining Cells

Bone lining cells are flat, elongated, inactive cells, localized in bone surfaces. Their function rests unknown, although some speculations exist. For example, these cells may be precursors for osteoblasts. They are also thought to be responsible for transfers of minerals, or even initiate the bone remodeling process in the presence of a mechanical or chemical stimulus.

1.3. Porosity and Bone

Porosity is an important feature of bone. It can be defined as the volume fraction of soft tissue. At the same time that bone can present a very high degree of porosity in some anatomical landmarks, it can have a very low degree in others. This peculiarity gives rise to a well-known classification: the trabecular (cancellous), with porosity ranging from 75% to 95%, and compact (cortical) bone, with porosity from 5% to 10%. The main differences between trabecular and compact bone rely on structure and functionality. While compact bone is mainly responsible for mechanical functions and protection, the trabecular bone shows a metabolic role.

Trabecular bone can be found in the ends of long bones (epiphysis), flat and cuboidal bones (Figure 1.4). The non-calcified regions are filled with marrow. Table 1.1 shows some microarchitectural and density parameters from human trabecular bone, measured with a high-resolution synchrotron radiation (SR p-CT) microtomography. In Figure 1.5 the three-dimensional (3D) microarchitecture reconstruction of trabecular bones with different degrees of porosities can be observed.

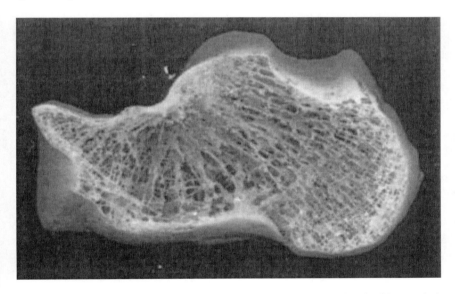

Figure 1.4. Trabecular (cancellous) bone in human calcaneus (Reprinted with permission from The Journal of the Acoustical Society of America, vol. 110, n. 6, Keith Wear, Fundamental precision limitations for measurements of frequency dependence of backscatter: Applications in tissue-mimicking phantoms and trabecular bone, p. 3280, Copyright (2001), Acoustic Society of America).

Table 1.1. Microarchitectural and density parameters from human trabecular bone, using SR p-CT microtomography (age ranging from 45 to 95 years)

Parameter	Mean	Standard deviation
Bone surface over total surface (BS/BV) [mm^{-1}]	25.78	4.59
Bone volume over total volume (BV/TV) [%]	11.50	5.52
Trabecular thickness (Tb.Th) [µm]	138.44	25.60
Trabecular spacing (Tb.Sp) [µm]	723.31	277.87
Degree of mineralization of bone (DMB) [g/cm^3]	1.08	0.03
Bone mineral density (BMD) [g/mm3]	123.70	56.00

From Padilla et al. (2008).

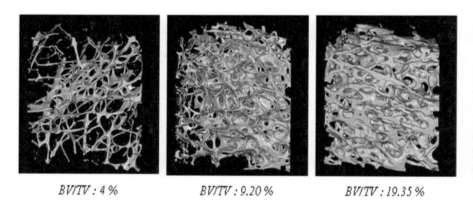

BV/TV : 4 %   *BV/TV : 9.20 %*   *BV/TV : 19.35 %*

Figure 1.5. 3D reconstruction of trabecular bone from high-resolution synchrotron radiation (SR p-CT) microtomography with different bone volume/total volume fractions (Reprinted from Bone, vol. 42, n. 6, F. Padilla, F. Jenson, V. Bousson, F. Peyrin, P. Laugier, Relationships of trabecular bone structure with quantitative ultrasound parameters: In vitro study on human proximal femur using transmission and backscatter measurements, p. 1196, Copyright (2008) with permission from Elsevier).

Compact bone forms the bone cortex (the name *cortical bone* comes from this). It forms the shaft of long bones and the shell of cancellous bone. A dense network of packed collagen fibrils forms concentric lamellae, and fibrils run in perpendicular planes (plywood-like arrangement) in adjacent lamellae (Figure 1.6). Canals with approximately 50 µm of diameter aligned to the long bones form the Haversian system, or Haversian canals, containing nerves and blood vessels. They are connected by Volkmann's canals, transverse to Haversian canals.

Bone Tissue Histology and Biology 11

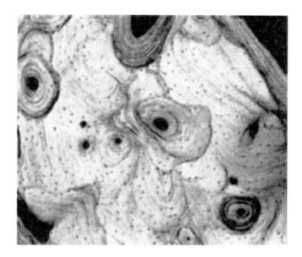

Figure 1.6. An image of cortical bone using a 400 MHz acoustic microscopy. It is possible to identify Haversian canals and contiguous circumferential lamellae (Reprinted with permission from The Journal of the Acoustical Society of America, vol. 115, n. 5, Emmanuel Bossy, Maryline Talmant, Pascal Laugier, Three-dimensional simulations of ultrasonic axial transmission velocity measurement on cortical bone models, p. 2316, Copyright (2004), Acoustic Society of America).

Bone structure is dynamic. Porosity may differ because of age, tissue remodeling or pathology. Figure 1.7(a) shows a cortical bone of a woman at the age of 55, and in (b) at the age of 90, the latter presenting a greater degree of porosity (Bossy et al., 2004). The same pattern can be observed in trabecular bone.

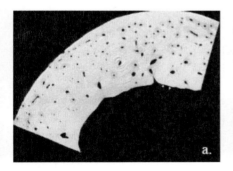 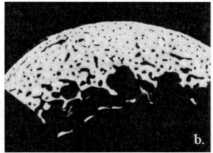

Figure 1.7. Cortical bone of a woman with (a) 55 years old; and (b) 90 years old (Courtesy from Dr. Emmanuel Bossy - Institut Langevin, ESPCI ParisTech, Paris, France).

The compact bone can be classified as primary and secondary bones. **Primary bone** is mineralized tissue deposited on an existing bone surface (for instance, the periosteum). The primary osteon and Haversian canal are formed in this way (circumferential lamellar bone). Another type of primary bone, the plexiform bone, consists of woven and lamellar bone mixed together to produce an appearance of a "brick wall". On the other hand there is the **secondary bone**, produced by a process known as bone remodeling, in which secondary osteons (Haversian systems) appear under the primary bone.

1.3.1. The Lamellar and the Woven Bone

From a microscopic point of view, it is possible to identify another level of organization: the lamellar bone and the woven bone.

The **lamellar bone** is a tissue with a high level of organization. The lamellae are parallel layers formed by collagen fibers and mineral crystals, giving the anisotropic characteristic of bone. The mineralization process occurs by using collagen as a "template". A layer of osteoid (unmineralized matrix) is always present on the surface under the osteoblasts. The deposit of mineral matrix can be made toward bone surface, or even surrounding the osteoblast to produce osteocytes.

Nevertheless, **woven bone** is poorly organized, with collagen fibers and crystals randomly arranged. The formation of this type of bone is very quick, however it is weaker than lamellar bone.

1.4. Bone Development

The ossification takes place by two basic phenomena: the intramembranous (or direct) ossification and the endochondral (or indirect) ossification.

Intramembranous ossification occurs during embryonic development. Bones of calvaria, some facial bones, and some parts of the mandible and clavicle develop essentially using this process, in which mesenchymal cells transform directly into osteoblasts. These cells migrate to produce initially types III, V and XI collagen, and finally the main protein component of bone, collagen type I. Sutures link the edges of bones when the growth is finished.

Another bone development process is the **endochondral ossification** which forms bones acting in joints. Hyaline cartilage tissue is produced from the recruitment, proliferation and differentiation of the embryonic mesenchymal cells, then progressively mineralized and replaced by bone. Proliferation of chondrocytes and its consequent hypertrophy occur in the direction of bone growth. It can be observed spicules of calcified cartilage below these cells, surrounded by osteoblasts. During this process a marrow cavity is formed with blood vessels, hematopoietic tissue, osteprogenitor cells and osteoblasts. The perichondrium surrounds the hyaline cartilage, and the periosteum surrounds the marrow cavity in the new formed bone, with peripheral osteoblasts bringing blood supply for the turnover of the bone (Jee, 2009).

Both intramembranous and endochondral ossifications (Figure 1.8) can be present in fracture healing, which will be discussed in Chapter 3.

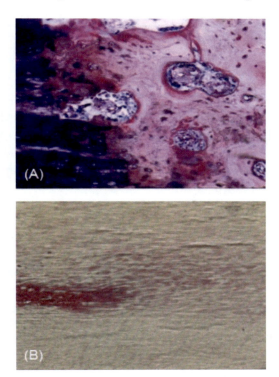

Figure 1.8. Endochondral and intramembranous ossification. In endochondral ossification (A), it can be seen the calcification of cartilage and subsequent replacement by bone tissue. In intramembranous ossification, mineralization takes place directly by osteoblasts (B) (Reprinted from Progress in Biophysics & Molecular Biology, vol. 93, Lutz Claes, Bettina Willie, The enhancement of bone regeneration by ultrasound, p. 388, Copyright (2007) with permission from Elsevier).

1.5. Cartilage

It is impossible to describe bone tissue biology and development without talking about cartilage tissue. This type of tissue is essential for endochondral ossification (in which long bones, the spine and ribs grow from a cartilage model and consequent bone formation) and for fracture regeneration (Chapter 3). It is also present in human body joints, ear, nose, bronchial tubes and intervertebral disks.

Body joints need a bearing surface made of cartilage. This articular cartilage contains no blood vessels or nerves. It is a flexible tissue composed of cells called **chondroblasts** (cells that produce the extracellular matrix) and the **chondrocytes** (chodroblasts caught in the matrix) which lie in spaces called lacunae. Chondrocytes represent between 0.4 % and 2 % of the total cartilage volume, and they may exist in four forms: active cells for extracellular matrix production; inactive cells which can evolve for the active form or for necrosis; degenerated cells; and necrotic cells. Approximately 70% of all cartilage matrix is filled with water.

The extracellular matrix is mainly composed of type II collagen (40% to 70% of the dry weight) and proteoglycans (15% to 40% of the dry weight). Other types of collagen in articular cartilage are type VI (present in pericellular adhesion molecule), type IX (fibril association and type II stabilization), type X (in hypertrophic zone of growth plate) and type XI (important in fibril growth control).

Three types of cartilage exist in human body: (1) the **hyaline cartilage**, found in articular surfaces, anterior end of the ribs, tracheal rings and growth plates (nonmineralized region of growth near the end of developing bones), is the most prevalent type of cartilage in the body; (2) the **elastic cartilage**, found in external ear, epiglottis and Eustachian tubes, presents a greater elasticity than hyaline cartilage, because of the great amount of elastic fibers; and (3) the **fibrocartilage**, forming the pubic symphysis, intervertebral disks, and tendon-bone attachments.

1.5.1. Growth of Long Bones

The long bones in children and adolescents have a region at each end of the bone (metaphysis), called **epiphyseal plate** (or **physis**, or **growth plate**). It is formed by hyaline cartilage. Endochondral ossification takes place for the initial bone development and chondrocytes are in constant mitotic division.

The epiphyseal plate has a very specific morphology (zonal arrangement). First of all, the **resting zone**, where cells are irregularly scattered and in constant division to provide chondrocytes for the growth plate; the **proliferative zone**, with chondrocytes under constant division; the **hypertrophic zone**, where chondrocytes are matured and hypertrophied; and the **calcification zone**, when the degenerated chondrocytes are progressively calcified.

As the maturing of the child's bones progresses, the epiphyseal plates are no longer necessary. The ossification of this region creates an epiphyseal line, and bone stops its growth (Figure 1.9).

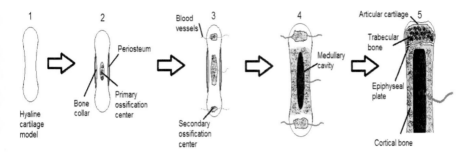

Figure 1.9. Growth of long bones: (1) the process initiates with a hyaline cartilage model; (2) a primary ossification center is formed, as well as the bone collar and periosteum; (3) secondary ossification centers are developed in epiphysis regions, and angiogenesis takes place; (4) a medullary cavity containing marrow tissue appears; (5) in children and adolescents, it is possible to observe the epiphyseal plate, as well as the trabecular bone in epiphysis and cortical bone in diaphysis.

Conclusion

This chapter brought brief information about bone tissue biology and histology. It was possible to understand how bone tissue develops, the metabolic role of each cell, structural features and the importance of cartilage in this context.

There was no intention here to completely explore this subject. Nowadays much more is known about bones, and much more is under intense research. The idea is to present a theoretical basis for the comprehension of ultrasound interaction with bone tissue, discussed in details later. Further reading of the references used in this book is suggested.

Bone tissue continues to be the main theme in the next two chapters. In Chapter 2, a biomechanical approach is presented, and in Chapter 3, fracture healing will be discussed in details.

References

Bossy, E., Talmant, M., & Laugier, P. (2004). Three-dimensional simulations of ultrasonic axial transmission velocity measurement on cortical bone models. *The Journal of the Acoustical Society of America, 115*, 2314-2324.

Bossy, E., Talmant, M., Peyrin, F., Akrout, L., Cloetens, P., & Laugier, P. (2004). An in vitro study of the ultrasonic axial transmission technique at the radius: 1-MHz velocity measurements are sensitive to both mineralization and intracortical porosity. *Journal of Bone and Mineral Research, 19*, 1548-1556.

Carter, D.R., & Beaupré, G.S. (2001). *Skeletal Function and Form: Mechanobiology of Skeletal Development, Aging, and Regeneration* (1st edition). New York, NY: Cambridge University Press.

Claes, L., & Willie, B. (2007). The enhancement of bone regeneration by ultrasound. *Progress in Biophysics & Molecular Biology, 93*, 384-398.

Jee, W.S.S. (2009). Integrated Bone Tissue Physiology: Anatomy and Physiology. In S. C. Cowin (Ed.), *Bone Mechanics Handbook* (2nd edition, pp. 1-1 – 1-68). New York, NY: Informa Healthcare USA, Inc.

Majeska, R. J. (2009). Cell Biology of Bone. In S. C. Cowin (Ed.), *Bone Mechanics Handbook* (2nd edition, pp. 2-1 – 2-24). New York, NY: Informa Healthcare USA, Inc.

Marks, S.C., & Odgren, P.R. (2002). Structure and Development of the Skeleton. In: J. P. Bilezikian, L. G. Raisz, & G. A. Rodan (Eds.), *Principles of Bone Biology* (2nd edition, pp. 3-15). Burlington, MA: Elsevier Inc.

Martin, R. B., Burr, D. B., & Sharkey, N. A. (2010). *Skeletal Tissue Mechanics* (1st edition). New York, NY: Springer-Verlag.

Padilla, F., Jenson, F., Bousson, V., Peyrin, F., & Laugier, P. (2008). Relationships of trabecular bone structure with quantitative ultrasound parameters: In vitro study on human proximal femur using transmission and backscatter measurements. *Bone, 42*, 1193-1202.

Rho, J.Y., Kuhn-Spearing, L., & Zioupos, P. (1998). Mechanical properties and the hierarchical structure of bone. *Medical Engineering & Physics, 20*, 92-102.

Wear, K. (2001). Fundamental precision limitations for measurements of frequency dependence of backscatter: Applications in tissue-mimicking phantoms and trabecular bone. *The Journal of the Acoustical Society of America, 110*, 3275-3282.

Chapter 2

Bone Tissue Mechanics

Abstract

Bone is a complex living solid with the ability to adapt its structure to the imposed loadings. For this reason, the study of solid mechanics is of utmost importance. There is a linear relationship between load and deformation until a point called proportional limit, with reduction of the curve's slope. After the yield point, a permanent deformation is produced (plastic deformation) and fractures can occur with increasing load. Some important mechanical concepts are: strength, which is defined as the load at the yield or fracture point; stiffness, which is the necessary load to deform a material; stress, which is the load per unit area; and strain, a measure of deformation. Essential parameters to characterize the mechanical properties are the Young's modulus, Poisson ratio, bulk and shear moduli, and shear strain. Bone can be modeled as an anisotropic, linear elastic solid. More specifically, bone has a special kind of anisotropy called orthotropy (the mechanical properties differ according to orthogonal directions). The Hook's law can be used to linearly relate the deformation (strain) to the force applied (stress). As cortical and trabecular bone present different structural patterns, it is expected that they also show different mechanical properties.

2.1. Introduction

If we talk about acoustics (specifically ultrasound for this book), we shall take a look in materials mechanics. **Solid mechanics** is a branch of mechanics concerning the behavior of solid materials under external actions (e.g., forces, displacements, temperature). The acoustical waves are time-varying deformations in a material medium, which is composed of atoms. Acoustics is concerned with material particles small enough to be forced into vibrational motion about its equilibrium position.

Bone is a complex living structure, which has an important feature: the ability to adapt its structure to the imposed loadings. The resulting structure from this adaptation is influenced by several mechanical principles. A first and well-accepted description of this dynamic behavior was made by a German anatomist named Julius Wolff (1836–1902). He stated that bone in a healthy vertebrate will adapt to the loads it is submitted during life. Bone strength will increase if loading on a particular bone increases, and the converse is true. The trabecular architecture can undergo adaptive changes, as well as the external cortical bone.

In the present chapter, the basis of solid mechanics is explored, as well as the biomechanics of bone tissue, providing background information that will be very useful in subsequent chapters of this book.

2.2. Basics of Solid Mechanics

2.2.1. Mechanical Equilibrium

An object is said to be in equilibrium if it is not moving or moving with constant velocity. This object is submitted to a system of N forces $\vec{F}_i$. We then consider in bold letters the vectors $\vec{F}_1$, $\vec{F}_2$, ..., $\vec{F}_N$. According the second law of Newton, it is said that the sum of these forces is zero, i.e., and the condition of force equilibrium is satisfied with

$$\sum_{i=1}^{N} \vec{F}_i = \vec{F}_1 + \vec{F}_2 + ... + \vec{F}_N = 0 \qquad (2.1)$$

A complete equilibrium demands a condition of moment equilibrium. Considering another system of vectors $\vec{R}_i$ ($\vec{R}_1$, $\vec{R}_2$, ..., $\vec{R}_N$), from a selected point to the point of the applied force $\vec{F}_i$, the moment of the force $\vec{F}_i$ with respect to the selected point will be the cross product of $\vec{R}_i$ with $\vec{F}_i$, and the sum of all the moments would be

$$\sum_{i=1}^{N} \vec{R}_i \vec{F}_i = \vec{R}_1 \vec{F}_1 + \vec{R}_2 \vec{F}_2 + ... + \vec{R}_N \vec{F}_N \qquad (2.2)$$

According to Cowin (2009), the **mechanical equilibrium** is reached when, for a set of couples $\vec{C}_k$ ($\vec{C}_1, \vec{C}_2, ..., \vec{C}_M$) we have

$$\sum_{i=1}^{N} \vec{R}_i \vec{F}_i + \sum_{k}^{M} \vec{C}_k = 0 \qquad (2.3)$$

2.2.2. Some Important Concepts

Two of the most important mechanical concepts are strength and stiffness. To understand the meaning of them, it is important to know how these variables can be estimated, using a test called **load-deformation**.

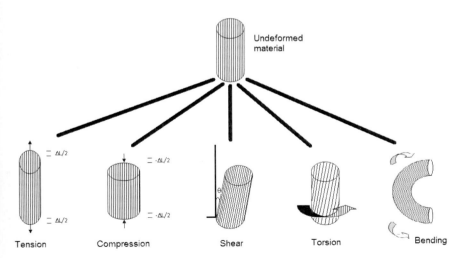

Figure 2.1. Possible deformations in a solid material: tension, compression, shear, torsion and bending.

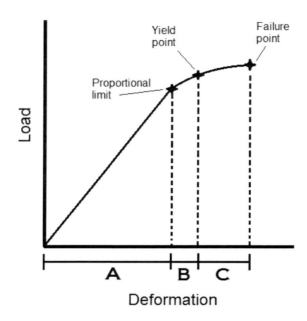

Figure 2.2. Typical load vs. deformation curve for a solid material. In A and B, the material is under linear and nonlinear elastic deformation, respectively. Region C represents plastic deformation (the material is permanently deformed).

The studied material is loaded in a desired manner (tension, compression, torsion, bending, shear, as seen in Figure 2.1) (Cullinane & Einhorn, 2002) and its deformation is recorded as a function of the applied load. There is a linear relationship between load and deformation until a point called proportional limit, in which the slope of the curve is reduced. The material presents a permanent deformation after the yield point (plastic deformation). With increasing load after this threshold, the ultimate load may be attained, and in some materials a fracture occurs (the failure point) (Figure 2.2).

The **strength** of a material can be defined as the load at the yield or fracture point (depending on the material or on the analysis being made); **stiffness** (or rigidity) may be the necessary load to deform it. Another parameter, the **compliance**, is the reciprocal of stiffness, and it means the ease to deform the material (Martin et al., 2010).

Other two important definitions are stress and strain. **Stress** is a measure of the internal forces acting within a deformable material, or simply the load per unit area. Figure 2.3 better presents this concept. Considering an axially loaded body (with an uniformly distributed load), the normal stress σ (in MPa) can be obtained using the equation

$$\sigma = \frac{F_n}{A} \tag{2.4}$$

where F_n is the normal force, perpendicularly applied to a given area A. There is also the so called shear stress (τ), when the force F_s occurs in shear (also shown in Figure 2.3), similarly calculated using the equation

$$\tau = \frac{F_s}{A} \tag{2.5}$$

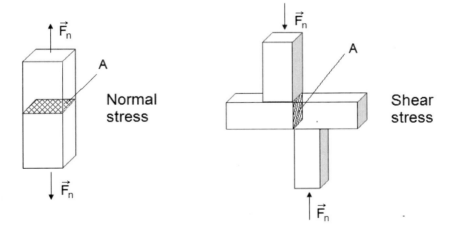

Figure 2.3. Schematic representations of normal (σ) and shear (τ) stress applied to area A.

Strain (ε) is simply a measure of deformation: it is the relative displacement between particles in a body. It can be calculated using the equation

$$\varepsilon = \frac{\Delta l}{l_0} \tag{2.6}$$

where Δl is the measured displacement, and l_0 is the initial body length.

A relation between stress and strain gives rise to another parameter called **elasticity** (E in MPa), and it is simply given by

$$E = \frac{\sigma}{\varepsilon} \tag{2.7}$$

also known as Young's modulus (or modulus of elasticity). Analyzing the load-deformation curve, it can be shown that the Young's modulus is the slope of the linear region.

The **Poisson ratio** (υ) is the ratio between the transverse strain component and the longitudinal strain component, then

$$\upsilon = -\frac{\varepsilon_t}{\varepsilon_l} \tag{2.8}$$

where ε_t is the transverse strain, and ε_l is the longitudinal strain.

An ordinary material may present $\upsilon < 0.5$, and for incompressible materials, $\upsilon = 0.5$.

There are other two important parameters to characterize the mechanical behavior of a solid medium. First, the **bulk modulus** (K), in MPa, which can be defined using the equation

$$K = -V \frac{\partial P}{\partial V} \tag{2.9}$$

where V is volume and P is pressure. This modulus can be also obtained with the relation

$$K = \frac{E}{3(1-2\upsilon)} \tag{2.10}$$

Finally, the **shear modulus** (G, also in MPa), which may be estimated using the equation

$$G = \frac{\tau}{\gamma} \quad (2.11)$$

where γ is the **shear strain**. Again, the Young's modulus and the Poisson's ratio can be used to calculate the shear modulus, using the equation

$$G = \frac{E}{2(1+\upsilon)} \quad (2.12)$$

2.2.3. The Hooke's Law

Bone can be modeled as an anisotropic, linear elastic solid. **Anisotropic** materials possess different mechanical properties for different directions of analysis. On the other hand, in **isotropic** bodies, mechanical properties are directionally independent. It can be said that bone has a special kind of anisotropy called **orthotropy**, which means that mechanical properties differ according to orthogonal directions (Mitton et al., 2011).

The Hooke's law can be used as a constitutive equation, and it says that the deformation (strain) is linearly proportional to the force applied (stress), and vice-versa. Generally speaking, the linear elastic equation may be represented by

$$\sigma_i = C_{ij}\varepsilon_j \quad (2.13)$$

where C is the stiffness tensor, a matrix with elastic constants C_{ij}. For an orthotropic material (bone, for example), the matrix C has nine independent coefficients:

$$[C] = \begin{bmatrix} C_{11} & C_{12} & C_{13} & 0 & 0 & 0 \\ C_{12} & C_{22} & C_{23} & 0 & 0 & 0 \\ C_{13} & C_{23} & C_{33} & 0 & 0 & 0 \\ 0 & 0 & 0 & C_{44} & 0 & 0 \\ 0 & 0 & 0 & 0 & C_{55} & 0 \\ 0 & 0 & 0 & 0 & 0 & C_{66} \end{bmatrix} \quad (2.14)$$

According to Cowin (2009), an orthotropic symmetry can be characterized by three perpendicular planes of mirror symmetry. A symmetry coordinate system is formed with the normals to these planes, and one set of the nine coefficients, the so-called **technical elastic constants**, can be defined: three Young's moduli (E_1, E_2 and E_3), three shear moduli (G_{12}, G_{13} and G_{23}) and six Poisson's ratios (v_{23}, v_{32}, v_{13}, v_{31}, v_{12} and v_{21}). Then, the following expression (compliance matrix and the technical constants) can be written:

$$\begin{bmatrix} \varepsilon_{11} \\ \varepsilon_{22} \\ \varepsilon_{33} \\ 2\varepsilon_{23} \\ 2\varepsilon_{13} \\ 2\varepsilon_{12} \end{bmatrix} = \begin{bmatrix} \frac{1}{E_1} & \frac{-v_{12}}{E_1} & \frac{-v_{13}}{E_1} & 0 & 0 & 0 \\ \frac{-v_{21}}{E_2} & \frac{1}{E_2} & \frac{-v_{23}}{E_2} & 0 & 0 & 0 \\ \frac{-v_{31}}{E_3} & \frac{-v_{32}}{E_3} & \frac{1}{E_3} & 0 & 0 & 0 \\ 0 & 0 & 0 & \frac{1}{G_{23}} & 0 & 0 \\ 0 & 0 & 0 & 0 & \frac{1}{G_{13}} & 0 \\ 0 & 0 & 0 & 0 & 0 & \frac{1}{G_{12}} \end{bmatrix} \begin{bmatrix} \sigma_{11} \\ \sigma_{22} \\ \sigma_{33} \\ \sigma_{23} \\ \sigma_{13} \\ \sigma_{12} \end{bmatrix} \quad (2.15)$$

For the transverse isotropic case, only 5 independent coefficients will be needed, because $E_1 = E_2$, $v_{12} = v_{21}$, $v_{31} = v_{32} = v_{13} = v_{23}$, $G_{23} = G_{31}$, and $G_{12} = E_1/2(1+ v_{12})$. Table 2.1 shows the elastic constants C_{ij} values for bovine and human cortical bone.

Table 2.1. Elastic constants C_{ij} for bovine (Lasaygues and Pithioux, 2002) and human (Van Buskirk and Ashman, 1981) cortical bone

C_{ij} (in GPa)	Bovine	Human
C_{11}	23.50	20.00
C_{22}	26.00	21.70
C_{33}	34.60	30.00
C_{44}	9.20	6.56
C_{55}	6.00	5.85
C_{66}	6.05	4.74
C_{12}	6.55	10.90
C_{13}	8.35	11.50
C_{23}	8.20	11.50

2.3. Mechanical Properties of Bone

According to Martin et al. (2010, p. 139), the mechanical properties of bone "represent a compromise between the need for stiffness to make muscle actions efficient, the need for compliance to absorb energy and avoid fracture, and the need for minimal skeletal weight". Indeed these three functions (muscle insertion, fracture resistance and relative low weight) must be harmonically performed by bone tissue.

Not every bone in our body will present the same mechanical properties. A simple explanation is that not every bone has the same function, or the same anatomical site. It is well known that bone remodeling is influenced by several events during life, mainly due to mechanical loadings. For this reason, for example, the cortical and the trabecular bone present different mechanical characteristics.

2.3.1. Cortical Bone

As it has already been said, cortical (or compact) bone forms the diaphyses of long bones and the shell of cancellous bone. Some typical cortical mechanical properties in humans are shown in Table 2.2 (for adult femur and tibia).

The mechanical properties of cortical bone are influenced by the osteons by three mechanisms (Martin et al., 2010):

- Continuous replacement of mineralized bone matrix with less calcified material;
- Increase of cortical porosity;
- Introduction of cement line interfaces.

Different types of osteons present different mechanical properties. Three classifications of osteons may be recognized, according to collagen fiber orientations: types L, A and T. Important studies of Ascenzi and Bonucci (1968, 1972) showed that osteons can adapt themselves individually according to loading demands during life. Table 2.3 shows the elastic modulus for different types of osteons.

Table 2.2. Some mechanical properties for human cortical bone (adult femur and tibia)

Parameter	Value (human)
Longitudinal elastic modulus (GPa)	17.4
Transverse elastic modulus (GPa)	9.6
Shear modulus (GPa)	3.51
Poisson's ratio	0.39
Longitudinal tensile yield stress (MPa)	115
Longitudinal compressive yield stress (MPa)	182
Transverse compressive yield stress (MPa)	121
Shear yield stress (MPa)	54
Longitudinal tensile ultimate stress (MPa)	133
Transverse tensile ultimate stress (MPa)	51
Longitudinal compressive ultimate stress (MPa)	195
Transverse compressive ultimate stress (MPa)	133
Shear ultimate stress (MPa)	69
Longitudinal tensile ultimate strain	0.029
Transverse tensile ultimate strain	0.032
Longitudinal compressive ultimate strain	0.022
Transverse compressive ultimate strain	0.046
Shear ultimate strain	0.33

From Cowin (1989)

Table 2.3. Elastic modulus values for different types of osteons (human femur)

Loading	Type of osteon	Elastic modulus (GPa)
Tension	Type L	11.7
	Type A	5.5
	Type T	-
Compression	Type L	6.3
	Type A	7.4
	Type T	9.3
Shear	Type L	3.3
	Type A	4.1
	Type T	4.1

From Ascenzi and Bonucci (1968, 1972)

The bone is an orthotropic material, i.e., the mechanical properties differ according to orthogonal directions. In order to provide a parameter to estimate anisotropy, the percentage compressive and shear elastic anisotropy were proposed, respectively Ac% and As%. These parameters are calculated using the expressions (Katz, 2008)

$$Ac\% = 100\frac{K^V - K^R}{K^V + K^R} \qquad (2.16)$$

$$As\% = 100\frac{G^V - G^R}{G^V + G^R} \qquad (2.17)$$

where K^V and K^R are the Voigt and Reuss bulk moduli, respectively, and G^V and G^R are the Voigt and Reuss shear moduli, respectively. For the transverse isotropic case, the Voigt moduli is given by

$$K^V = \frac{2(C_{11} + C_{12}) + 4(C_{13} + C_{33})}{9} \qquad (2.18)$$

and

$$G^V = \frac{(C_{11} + C_{12}) - 4C_{13} + 2C_{33} + 12(C_{44} + C_{66})}{30} \qquad (2.19)$$

and the Reuss moduli is given by

$$K^R = \frac{C_{33}(C_{11} + C_{12}) - 2C_{13}^2}{(C_{11} + C_{12} - 4C_{13} + 2C_{33})} \qquad (2.20)$$

and

$$G^R = \frac{5[C_{33}(C_{11} + C_{12}) - 2C_{13}^2]C_{44}C_{66}}{2\{[C_{33}(C_{11} + C_{12}) - 2C_{13}^2](C_{44} + C_{66}) + [C_{44}C_{66}(2C_{11} + C_{12}) + 4C_{13} + C_{33}]/3\}} \qquad (2.21)$$

for the orthotropic case, the Voigt moduli may be calculated by

$$K^V = \frac{C_{11} + C_{22} + C_{33} + 2(C_{12} + C_{13} + C_{23})}{9} \qquad (2.22)$$

and

$$G^V = \frac{[C_{11}+C_{22}+C_{33}+3(C_{44}+C_{55}+C_{66})-(C_{12}+C_{13}+C_{23})]}{15}$$

(2.23)

and the Reuss moduli will be given by

$$K^R = \frac{\Delta}{C_{11}C_{22}+C_{22}C_{33}+C_{33}C_{11}} - 2(C_{11}C_{23}+C_{22}C_{13}+C_{33}C_{12})$$ (2.24)
$$+ 2(C_{12}C_{23}+C_{23}C_{13}+C_{13}C_{12})-(C_{12}^2+C_{13}^2+C_{23}^2)$$

and

$$G^R = 15/(4\{(C_{11}C_{22}+C_{22}C_{33}+C_{33}C_{11}+C_{11}C_{23}+C_{22}C_{13}+C_{33}C_{22})$$ (2.25)

$$-[C_{12}(C_{12}+C_{23})+C_{23}(C_{23}+C_{13})+C_{13}(C_{13}+C_{12})]\}/\Delta + 3(1/C_{44}+1/C_{55}+1/C_{66}))$$

where Δ is a matrix given by

$$\Delta = \begin{bmatrix} C_{11} & C_{12} & C_{13} \\ C_{12} & C_{22} & C_{23} \\ C_{13} & C_{23} & C_{33} \end{bmatrix}$$

(2.26)

Table 2.4 shows Ac% and As% values for various types of bone.

Table 2.4. Percentage compressive (Ac%) and shear (As%) elastic anisotropy for various types of bones

Specimen	Ac%	As%
Bovine femur[a]	1.52	2.07
Human femur[b]	1.04	1.05
Human femur[a]	1.50	1.88
Haversian system[c]	1.08	0.77

[a] Van Buskirk and Ashman (1981)
[b] Yoon and Katz (1976)
[c] Katz and Meunier (1987)

The mechanical properties of cortical and osteonal bone may also be affected by another seven factors (Martin et al., 2010):

Porosity: is the ratio of void volume to total volume. It is expected that bone strength decreases as porosity increases. In cortical and trabecular bone, the mechanical properties are affected by the Haversian system and marrow cavities, respectively. Several relationships between Young's modulus (E) and porosity (p) have been proposed. For example, the equation found by Currey (1988) is presented here,

$$E = 23.4(1-p)^{5.74} \qquad (2.27)$$

- Mineralization degree: bone mechanical properties are affected by the tissue mineralization degree. The volumetric mineralization (amount of mineral per unit volume of whole bone) is influenced by the porosity and mineralization of the bone matrix. However the specific mineralization (amount per volume of bone matrix) is not a function of porosity.
- Density: the term apparent density (ρ_a) is the most applied term for bone tissue, and it is the mass of a volume divided by its total volume. It is known that the bone total volume (V_T) is the sum of the bony matrix volume (V_b) and the soft tissue (void) volume (V_v). The bone volume fraction (BVF) may be calculated using the expression :

$$BVF = \frac{V_b}{V_v} \qquad (2.28)$$

and porosity p may be given by

$$p = \frac{V_v}{V_T} \qquad (2.29)$$

Finally, we can calculate the apparent density ρ_a (in g/cm^3) using the expression

$$\rho_a = \rho_b - (\rho_b - \rho_v)p \qquad (2.30)$$

where ρ_b and ρ_V are the density of bone tissue and soft tissue, respectively. Values of 1.8 to 2.0 g/cm³ can be considered for cortical bone apparent density.

Researchers have been proposing relationships between the apparent density and Young's modulus. For example, Morgan et al. (2003) used the following equation to estimate E as a function of ρ_a

$$E = 8920\rho_a^{1.83} \tag{2.31}$$

- Architecture and collagen fiber orientation: internal architectures of bone affect mechanical properties. For example, primary lamellar bone is stronger than secondary lamellar bone. The collagen fiber orientation can also influence these properties, as it can be seen comparing the stronger lamellar bone (parallel collagen fibers) and woven bone (randomly oriented fibers).
- Microdamage: bone damage can occur because of loading above the yield stress, or even due to loading under the yield point during certain period of time (Mitton et al., 2011). Microdamage can affect bone properties, and it is related to the initial Young's modulus E_0 and the Young's modulus for the nth loading cycle E_n according to the equation

$$D = 1 - \frac{E_n}{E_0} \tag{2.32}$$

- Rate of deformation: considering that bone is a viscoelastic material, the rate of deformation can considerably affect its mechanical properties. Considering bone as an anisotropic linear viscoelastic material, one can describe the viscoelastic behavior using Boltzmann superposition integral equation (Katz, 2008)

$$\sigma_{ij}(t) = \int_{-\infty}^{t} C_{ijkl}(t-\tau) \frac{d\varepsilon_{kl}(\tau)}{d\tau} d\tau \tag{2.33}$$

where $\sigma_{ij}(t)$ and $\varepsilon_{kl}(\tau)$ are the second-rank stress and strain tensors, respectively. $C_{ijkl}(t-\tau)$ is the fourth-rank relaxation modulus tensor.

2.3.2. Trabecular Bone

Trabecular bone is found in the ends of long bones (epiphysis), flat and cuboidal bones. Non-calcified regions (void spaces) filled with marrow tissue can be macroscopically identified. Load-deformation curves in compression show that the void spaces collapse with a compaction of trabeculae. Therefore fractures into pieces are not observed in the case of trabecular bone.

The mechanical properties of trabecular bone can be affected by several aspects. The apparent density of trabecular bone is 1.0 to 1.4 g/cm^3. It presents a smaller mineral content and greater water content than in cortical bone. Lamellar orientation is also different. The anisotropy of trabecular bone can also influence the elastic modulus and strength.

It is a hard task to measure mechanical properties from trabecular bone since each trabecula presents small dimensions compared to cortical bone. According to Guo and Goldstein (1997), the reported Young's modulus for trabecular bone range from 0.76 to 20 GPa, depending on the measurement method (ultrasonic, nanoidentation, acoustic microscopy etc.), becoming a subject of controversy.

Table 2.5 presents values of Young's modulus found by many authors for trabecular bone. Note that there are different methods for elastic modulus estimation.

Table 2.5. Young's modulus for trabecular bone estimated by different methods

Method	Young's modulus (E) in GPa
Ultrasound[a]	14.8
Tensile test[a]	10.4
Nanoidentation[b]	19.4
Acoustic microscopy[c]	17.4

[a] Rho et al. (1993)
[b] Rho et al. (1999)
[c] Bumrerraj and Katz (2001)

Conclusion

This chapter aimed at generally presenting the basics of bone mechanics. First of all a theoretical background on solid mechanics was discussed, followed by a description of the mechanical properties of cortical and trabecular bone.

The knowledge of mechanical aspects of bone tissue is of utmost importance to understand the ultrasound propagation phenomena. Some further reading for a complete panorama can be recommended. -The books "Bone Mechanics Handbook" (ed. Stephen Cowin, 2009), and "Skeletal Tissue Mechanics" (R. Bruce Martin et al., 2010) are good examples.

The next chapter deals with the fracture healing phenomenon, a complex mechano-chemical event to reestablish bone continuity and function, and also a therapeutic target for ultrasound stimulation.

References

Ascenzi, A., & Bonucci, E. (1968). The compressive properties of single osteons. *Anatomical Record, 161,* 377-391.

Ascenzi, A., & Bonucci, E. (1972). The shearing properties of single osteons. *Anatomical Record, 172,* 499-510.

Bumrerraj, S., & Katz, J. L. (2001). Scanning acoustic microscopy study of human cortical and trabecular bone. *Annals of Biomedical Engineering, 29,* 1034-1042.

Cowin, S. C. (1989). *Bone Mechanics* (1st edition). Boca Raton, FL: CRC Press.

Cowin, S. C. (2009). Mechanics of Materials. In S. C. Cowin (Ed.), *Bone Mechanics Handbook* (2nd edition, pp. 6-1 – 6-24). New York, NY: Informa Healthcare USA, Inc.

Cullilane, D. M., & Einhorn, T. A. (2002). Biomechanics of Bone. In: J. P. Bilezikian, L. G. Raisz, & G. A. Rodan (Eds.), *Principles of Bone Biology* (2nd edition, pp. 3-15). Burlington, MA: Elsevier Inc.

Currey, J. D. (1988). The effect of porosity and mineral content on the Young's modulus of elasticity of compact bone. *Journal of Biomechanics, 21,* 131-139.

Guo, X. E., Goldstein, S. A. (1997). Is trabecular bone tissue different from cortical bone tissue? *Forma, 12,* 185-196.

Katz, J. L., & Meunier, A. (1980). The elastic anisotropy of bone. *Journal of Biomechanics, 20,* 1063-1070.

Katz, J. L. (2008). Mechanics of Hard Tissue. In D. R. Peterson, & J. D. Bronzino (Eds.), *Biomechanics: Principles and Applications* (1st edition, pp. 1-2 – 1-20). Boca Raton, FL: CRC Press.

Lasaygues, P., & Pithioux, M. (2002). Ultrasonic characterization of orthotropic elastic bovine bones. *Ultrasonics, 39,* 567-573.

Martin, R. B., Burr, D. B., & Sharkey, N. A. (2010). *Skeletal Tissue Mechanics* (1st edition). New York, NY: Springer-Verlag.

Mitton, D., Roux, C., & Laugier, P. (2011). Bone Overview. In: P. Laugier, & G. Haïat (Eds.), *Bone Quantitative Ultrasound* (1st edition, pp. 1 - 28). New York, NY: Springer.

Morgan, E.F., Bayraktar, H.H., & Keaveny, T.M. (2003). Trabecular bone modulus–density relationships depend on anatomic site. *Journal of Biomechanics, 36*, 897–904.

Rho, J. Y., Ashman, R. B., & Turner, C. H. (1993). Young's modulus of trabecular and cortical bone material: ultrasonic and microtensile measurements. *Journal of Biomechanics, 26*, 111-119.

Rho, J. Y., Roy, M. E., Tsui, T. Y., & Pharr, G. M. (1999). Elastic properties of microstructural components of human bone tissue as measured by indentation. *Journal of Biomedical Materials Research, 45*, 48-54.

Van Buskirk, W. C., & Ashman R. B. (1981). The elastic moduli of bone. In: S.C. Cowin (Ed.), *Mechanical Properties of Bone AMD, 45*, pp. 131–143. New York, NY: American Society of Mechanical Engineers.

Yoon, H. S., & Katz, J. L. (1976). Ultrasonic wave propagation in human cortical bone - II. Measurements of elastic properties and microhardness. *Journal of Biomechanics, 9*, 459-464.

Chapter 3

The Fracture Healing Phenomenon

Abstract

Fracture healing is a sequence of biological events involving molecular signaling to reprise embryological development phases and restore bone continuity and function. Two types of fracture healing can be defined: the primary (or direct) and the secondary (or indirect) healing, the latter aiming at developing the callus tissue by means of intramembranous and endochondral ossifications. Three steps can be distinguished in fracture regeneration: inflammatory, reparative and remodeling phases. All healing phases depend on signaling molecules (for example, citokines, BMP's, TGF-β etc.) which regulate the activity and differentiation of important cells. Nowadays it is well established that tissue differentiation during callus formation may be affected by stress and strain invariants of hydrostatic stress and distortional stress (mechanobiology-dependence of fracture healing). Many researchers have been proposing numerical models to estimate parameters which influence tissue differentiation during fracture healing. Computational simulations using finite element analysis (FEA) use material properties taken from literature to predict the fracture healing process, giving new insights into this physiological phenomenon.

3.1. Introduction

As we have seen in the first two chapters, bone is a complex, specialized connective tissue, maintaining its elasticity even with the presence of a high mineralized extracellular matrix. When bone fracture occurs, an acute response takes place for bone induction called fracture healing, by means of molecular signaling which represents a multistage repair process presenting an organized temporal and spatial sequence.

A broken bone means that the tissue exceeded its mechanical capacity to support loading. Fractures can be classified as traumatic (very common occurrence in emergency rooms), and pathological fractures (which are caused by bone weakening diseases, for example, osteoporosis, osteomalacia, Paget's disease and tumors).

Severe complications can appear with a default in bone healing. Non-union (production of pseudoarthrosis, a jointlike structure made of cartilage), delayed unions and infections may bring important negative consequences for patients and a socioeconomic burden, particularly due to the high costs in health care (Kanararis and Giannoudis, 2007).

In this chapter, a brief theoretical background for fracture healing will be presented since it will be necessary for the comprehension of the mechanisms underlying ultrasound fracture healing stimulation and quantitative ultrasound fracture assessment.

3.2. Understanding Fracture Healing

Fracture healing is a well orchestrated phenomenon, a response for a disruption in bone continuity and integrity. When the bone is broken, a sequence of biological events involving molecular signaling takes place, in order to repeat some embryological development phases, like intramembranous and endochondral ossification.

Two types of fracture healing can be defined: the primary (or direct) and the secondary (or indirect) healing. The **primary fracture healing** consists in the formation of the so called **cutting cones**, which are simple remodeling units to reestablish bone continuity, with a direct new haversian system formation across the fracture line. There is no callus tissue in this situation. On the other hand, the **secondary fracture healing** corresponds to the combination of intramembranous and endochondral ossification (already

The Fracture Healing Phenomenon 39

discussed in Chapter 1). In this case, a **callus tissue** will be formed in an attempt to restore bone continuity, then facilitating the progress of the healing process.

Figure 3.1 provides a schematic illustration of callus formation and the direction of bone apposition, as well as histological sections of callus tissue from sheep metatarsal, showing intramembranous and endochondral ossifications (Claes and Heigele, 1999). Figure 3.2 shows the phases of callus tissue from the fracture line until the calcified callus.

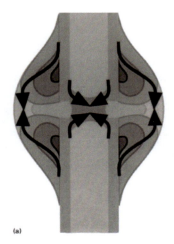
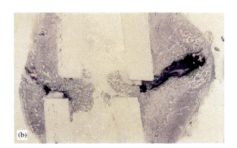
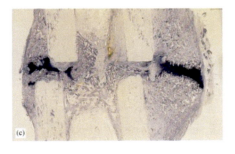

Figure 3.1. In (a) a schematic illustration of callus formation, with the arrows indicating the direction of bone apposition. In (b) and (c), histological sections from a sheep metatarsal callus tissue in which is possible to observe zones of fibrocartilage (colored violet) in the middle of the periosteal callus (endochondral ossification), and areas of intramembranous bone formation in the peripheral part of the periosteal callus and in the endosteal area (Reprinted from Journal of Biomechanics, vol. 32, n. 3, L. E. Claes, C. A. Heigele, Magnitudes of local stress and strain along bony surfaces predict the course and type of fracture healing, p. 255, Copyright (1999) with permission from Elsevier).

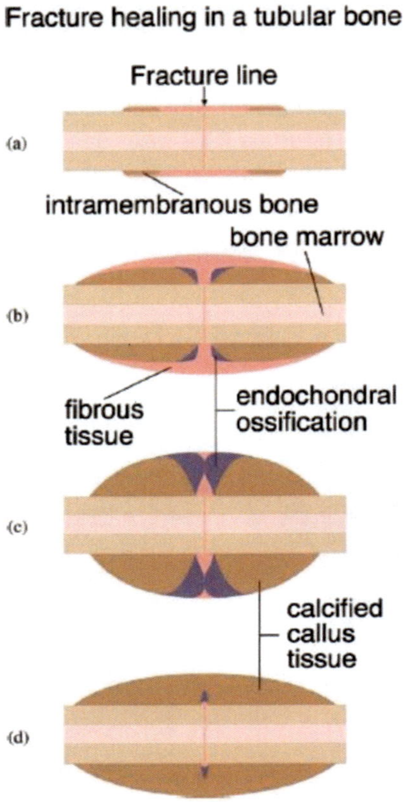

Figure 3.2. Phases of fracture healing in a tubular bone, showing the intramembranous and endochondral ossifications in callus tissue (Reprinted from Progress in Biophysics & Molecular Biology, vol. 93, Lutz Claes, Bettina Willie, The enhancement of bone regeneration by ultrasound, p. 389, Copyright (2007) with permission from Elsevier).

More generally speaking, fracture healing can be divided into three steps: inflammatory, reparative and remodeling phases (Martin et al., 2011):

- Inflammatory phase: the initial response for fracture healing is to immobilize the fracture line (by means of pain and local swelling) and assure the activation of osteogenic cells for reparation. A release of signaling molecules such as growth and differentiation factors, inflammatory cytokines and hormones recruits primary and mesenchymal cells to the injury site.

- Reparative phase: during this phase, the callus tissue is formed. An intense mesenchymal cells differentiation begins in parallel with a local vascular proliferation. Endochondral ossification takes place, as well as direct bone formation by osteoblasts. An inadequate immobilization can lead to deficient vascularization, and therefore a differentiation of stem cells in chondroblasts (which facilitates pseudoarthrosis generation) can be observed. If the regeneration process continues successfully, the callus is then progressively mineralized, becoming increasingly rigid (which is called bony or hard callus). When the rigidity of this callus equals or surpasses that of cortical bone, the reparative phase is finished.
- Remodeling phase: although bony callus has a great strength at this stage, the fracture site still presents a reduced efficiency. The remodeling phase restores the original geometrical contour and internal structure of fracture, to recover prior mechanical properties.

Figure 3.3 presents a comparison of typical fracture healing times (in weeks) for some upper and lower limb bones. It is known that some factors (Table 3.1) may compromise healing and delay the regeneration process. A **delayed union** is a healing not completed by 3 months, and some of these fractures may still remain unconsolidated at 9 months post-fracture (in this case called **nonunions**) (Hadjiargyrou et al., 1998).

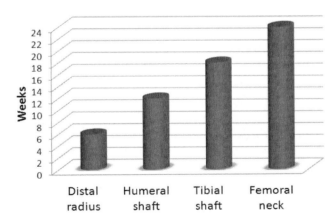

Figure 3.3. Typical fracture healing times for some upper and lower limbs bones (according to Martin et al., 2011).

Table 3.1. Possible causes of delayed union (Reprinted from Injury, vol. 39, Peter Siska, Gary Gruen, Hans Pape, External adjuncts to enhance fracture healing: What is the role of ultrasound?, p. 1097, Copyright (2008) with permission from Elsevier)

Local factors	Systemic factors
Blood supply to the bone	Patient age
Fracture location	Gender
Fracture type	Hormonal effects
Bone loss	Smoking
Open fracture	Diabetes
Post-operative infection	Alcoholism
Extent of soft tissue damage	
Fracture gap and soft tissue interposition	
Pre-reduction displacement	
Poor stabilization or fixation	

3.2.1. Molecular Signaling

All healing phases depend on signaling molecules. They regulate the activity and differentiation of several important cells. Some of these molecules are (Dimitriou et al., 2005; Phillips, 2005):

- Transforming growth factors β – TGFβ): released by platelets, inflammatory cells, endothelium, extracellular matrix, chondrocytes and osteoblasts. They are responsible for the stimulation of mesenchymal stem cells - MSC) in the early stages of bone regeneration;
- Bone morphogenetic proteins – BMPs): released by osteoprogenitors and mesenchymal cells, osteoblasts, extracellular matrix and chondrocytes. They promote differentiation of osteoprogenitors and mesenchymal cells into osteoblasts and chondrocytes, respectively and are present at various stages of healing;
- Fibroblast growth factors – FGF): released by macrophages, monocytes, mesenchymal cells, osteoblasts and chondrocytes. They stimulate angiogenesis and mitogenesis of mesenchymal and epithelial cells, osteoblasts and chondrocytes;
- Insulin like growth factors – IGF): released by bone matrix, endothelial and mesenchymal cells, and osteoblasts. They are responsible for proliferation and differentiation of osteoprogenitor

cells. IGF-1 is present during all healing phases, and IGF-2 acts during endochondral ossification;
- Platelet-derived growth factors – PDGF): released in initial stages of bone healing by platelets, macrophages, monocytes, endothelial cells and osteoblasts. They are mitogenic for mesenchymal cells and osteoblasts, and chemotactic for mesenchymal and inflammatory cells;
- Cytokines (interleukin-1, ou IL-1, IL-6, tumour necrosis factor-alpha – TNFα): released by mesenchymal cells, macrophages, and some inflammatory cells. They present a chemotactic effect on inflammatory cells. Besides that they recruit fibrogenic cells, promote angiogenesis and stimulate the synthesis of bone matrix. It is known that increased levels of cytokines are found in the first three days of healing and during bone remodeling;
- Metalloproteinases: bone extracellular matrix is their source. At the final stages of healing (including bone remodeling), the degradation of cartilage and bone is stimulated by them for the subsequent invasion of blood vessels;
- Vascular-endothelial growth factors – VEGF): they stimulate endothelial cell proliferation at endochondral ossification and bone formation;
- Angiopoietin: responsible for the formation of vessel structures, and present throughout the fracture healing process.

3.2.2. Mechanobiology of Bone Regeneration

Nowadays much is known about the effects of bone mechanobiology (which is the study of how mechanical conditions affect the bone biologic processes) in the proliferation and differentiation of bone cells during bone regeneration. However, there are still some controversies among scientists. Carter and Beaupré (2007, p. 162-163), two important researchers in this domain, stated the following reasons for that:

> The existence of different hypotheses concerning the influence of mechanical loading on tissue differentiation is not, for the most part, a consequence of conflicting biological observations. Much of the confusion has been a result of difficulties encountered in identifying and understanding the local physical environment. Many investigators have

misinterpreted or have given incomplete descriptions of the mechanical loading of the tissue under consideration, and many make no distinction between constant and intermittently applied loads.

Based on a number of *in vivo* experiments, the German researcher Friedrich Pauwels presented important concepts on bone mechanobiology, applying loads and verifying local stresses and strain levels. His ideas may be summarized as follows (Pauwels, 1980):

- Tissue differentiation may be affected by stress and strain invariants of hydrostatic stress and distortional stress;
- Distortional stresses result in elongation in one direction;
- In pseudoarthrosis and angulated fractures, there is a formation of parallel collagen fibers;
- Figure 3.4 depicts a schematic representation of Pauwels's view. Tissue deformation (or stretching) and high hydrostatic pressure (compression) produces collagen fibers (connective tissue) and cartilage tissue, respectively, from bone mesenchymal cells. A combination of deformation and compression would produce fibrocartilage.

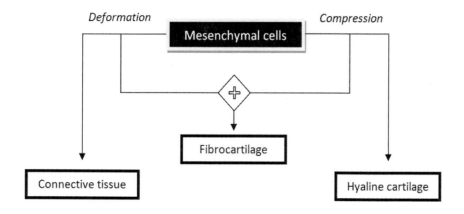

Figure 3.4. Schematic representation of Pauwels's view (Pauwels, 1980). Tissue deformation leads to connective tissue production. Compression produces hyaline cartilage tissue. A combination of deformation and compression produces fibrocartilage.

According to Pauwels's hypothesis, it could only be possible to form bone tissue after the mechanical stabilization of the fracture site, by the soft tissue reducing both deformation and compression stimuli.

Years later, Carter et al. (1998) contributed to this field with different ideas from Pauwels's point of view. They proposed a method to estimate local stress or strain history using cyclic tissue loading. A schematic representation of that can be seen in Figure 3.5. The lines that separate different tissue regions are "cutoff" values. The "tension line" indicates that fibrous tissue is formed above a certain level of principal strain, and the "pressure line" shows that cartilage may be formed below some critical level of hydrostatic pressure. If we are to the left of the pressure line, cartilage is formed and maintained due to a history of high hydrostatic pressure. However, if we are above the tension line, fibrous matrix is produced and maintained because of high tensile strain levels. The association of tensile strain and hydrostatic compression forms fibrocartilage. In regions where there is neither compressive nor tensile stimuli, direct bone formation takes place. Nevertheless, a key point for an adequate regeneration is blood supply. The production of bone matrix can be changed by cartilage formation where regions of low oxygen tension are found.

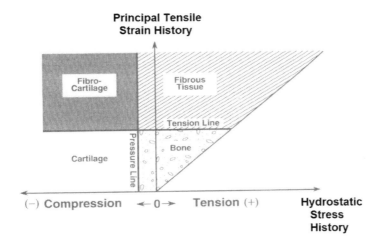

Figure 3.5. Illustration showing how hydrostatic stress history and maximal principal tensile strain history can influence the differentiation of mesenchymal tissue during bone regeneration (Reprinted from Dennis R. Carter & Gary S. Beaupré, *Skeletal Function and Form: Mechanobiology of Skeletal Development, Aging, and Regeneration*, p. 166, Copyright (2001) with permission from Cambridge University Press).

These theoretical approaches brought new possibilities. The emphasis on stress and strain history, and the application of cyclically applied loads, enabled the numerical modeling of the fracture healing phenomenon.

3.2.3. Nonrigid and Rigid Fixation

The therapeutic management for the majority of fractures is the **nonrigid fixation**, with the application of plaster casts to immobilize the affected limb, without the need for surgery. This approach allows some interfragmentary movements, which is important for callus formation. According to Carter & Beaupré (2007), a well-aligned transverse fracture presents axial compression, bending and torsion stimuli, and factors like fracture location, patient's activity and type of treatment will influence these loads. Then bone bridging takes place at the outer surface of callus, substantially increasing local stiffness. The endochondral ossification begins toward the fracture line, and it is highly affected by the mechanical stress history. Bone formation will depend directly on the intermittent loads during regeneration.

However, the **rigid fixation** corresponds to the use of implants (metal plates, screws) to stabilize the fracture site. Bone is directly formed from a callus with small dimensions and low quantity of fibrous tissue and fibrocartilage, due to an adequate vascularity and an almost complete fracture gap immobilization. This fixation can assure contact between bone fragments, enabling primary fracture healing (cutting cones).

3.3. Numerical Modeling of Fracture Healing

Many researchers have been proposing numerical models to estimate parameters which influence tissue differentiation during fracture healing. The hypothesis of Pauwels, Carter and co-workers gave some insight about the effect of interfragmentary movements modulating the healing process.

The numerical simulations (usually using the finite element analysis - FEA) generally applied some material properties (considering a linear poroelastic material, values taken from literature) for the tissue elements in the model. For example, the Young's modulus (MPa), permeability (m^4/Ns),

Poisson's ratio, fluid bulk modulus (MPa), solid bulk modulus (MPa) and porosity are parameters commonly used.

Carter et al. (1988, 1998) were the first to use FEA with a tissue differentiation algorithm to predict callus changes during bone regeneration. Claes and Heigele (1999) developed a model for fracture healing in which bone would be produced along the edges of existing calcified tissue, and tissue formation would depend on local stress and strain values. Another characteristic of their algorithm was the implementation of limits for when the different types of tissue differentiation would occur (intramembranous and endochondral ossification, formation of connective tissue).

Another algorithm considered that connective tissue is composed by fluid and solid phases (Prendergast, 1997; Lacroix and Prendergast, 2002), proposing two biophysical stimuli for each phase: deviatoric strain (solid phase) and fluid velocity (solid phase). According to them, high magnitudes of both deviatoric strain and fluid velocity lead to the formation of fibrous tissue, and low values of these parameters lead to ossification.

Four years later, Isaksson et al. (2006a) developed a finite element analysis study to compare these previous algorithms, and they hypothesized that tissue differentiation in fracture healing could be equally regulated by the individual mechanical stimuli: the deviatoric strain, the pore pressure and fluid velocity. They observed some small differences among the algorithms, and besides they found that deviatoric strain alone was able to simulate the tissue differentiation during normal fracture healing equally well as the other algorithms. The same group has tried to corroborate these mechanoregulatory models with histological data at 4 and 8 weeks after fracture (Isaksson et al., 2006b). The algorithm which was regulated by deviatoric strain and fluid velocity was the most accurate for torsional rotation *in vivo*. Figures 3.6 and 3.7 show, respectively, the interfragmentary movement and stiffness in the fracture gap during the healing process, and the predicted fracture healing pattern with torsional rotation, for each algorithm (Carter et al., Claes and Heigele, Lacroix and Prendergast, and deviatoric strain alone).

In 2008, the same group of Hanna Isaksson proposed a model which coupled cellular mechanisms to mechanical stimulation during fracture healing (Isaksson et al., 2008). In this model, mesenchymal cells, fibroblasts, chondrocytes and osteoblasts proliferated, differentiated, migrated and produced an extracellular matrix, based on mechanical stimuli. It was then possible to calculate extracellular matrices of connective tissue, cartilage and bone. The results of three loads on the predicted cell concentrations in the immediate fracture gap are depicted in Figure 3.8.

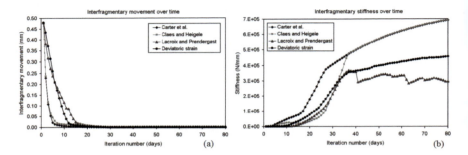

Figure 3.6. Results from the study of Isaksson et al. (2006a). The interfragmentary movement (a) and the interfragmentary stiffness (b) in the fracture gap during the healing process, for each analyzed algorithm (Reprinted from Journal of Biomechanics, vol. 39, Hanna Isaksson, Woulter Wilson, Corrinus van Donkelaar, Rik Huiskes, Keita Ito, Comparison of biophysical stimuli for mechano-regulation of tissue differentiation during fracture healing, p. 1513, Copyright (2006) with permission from Elsevier).

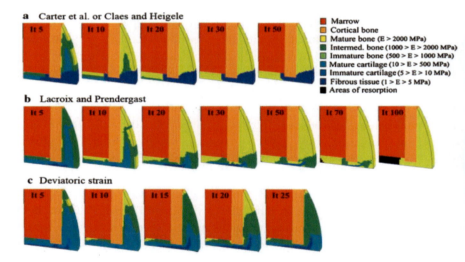

Figure 3.7. Results from simulations of Isaksson et al. (2006b) showing patterns of fracture healing for each algorithm. Different colors represent different types of tissues in the model (marrow, cortical bone, mature and immature bone, intermediate bone, mature and immature cartilage, fibrous tissue and areas of resorption) (Reprinted from Journal of Orthopaedic Research, vol. 24, Hanna Isaksson, Corrinus van Donkelaar, Rik Huiskes, Keita Ito, Corroboration of mechanoregulatory algorithms for tissue differentiation during fracture healing: comparison with in vivo results, p. 904, Copyright (2006) with permission from John Wiley and Sons).

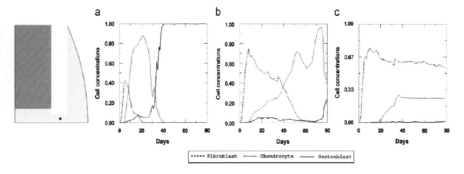

Figure 3.8. Results on the predicted cell concentrations in the immediate fracture for (a) 300 N load; (b) 400 N load; and (c) 500 N load (Reprinted from Journal of Theoretical Biology, vol. 252, Hanna Isaksson, Corrinus van Donkelaar, Rik Huiskes, Keita Ito, A mechano-regulatory bone-healing model incorporating cell-phenotype specific activity, p. 240, Copyright (2008) with permission from Elsevier).

More recently, Byrne et al. (2011) simulated the fracture healing process in human tibia, using a discrete lattice modeling approach. A mechanoregulation algorithm was also used to model cells proliferation, migration, apoptosis and differentiation. Simulations were run with a realistic anatomical 3D geometry and muscle loading, providing evidences that simulations could be used in pre-operative planning.

Conclusion

Chapter 3 presented a theoretical framework for fracture healing, and a pathobiological process that takes place following a fracture, in order to restore mechanical stability and function. More than a simple gap restoration, this phenomenon encompasses a complex cascade of chemical reactions and chemotactic signaling.

Recent applications of computational simulations coupled with experimental methodologies have aided researchers worldwide to develop new hypothesis concerning fracture healing. This approach has become possible with increasing scientific knowledge about molecular biology and informatics, enabling the prediction of spatial and temporal alterations in callus tissue during the regeneration process. However great challenges are still ahead. Many of the processes underlying fracture regeneration are unknown. Besides, it is not yet well established which are the most important input parameters to be used in the models. For a more detailed and comprehensive reading, the book "Skeletal Function and Form: Mechanobiology of Skeletal Development, Aging, and Regeneration" (Carter and Beaupré, 2001) is recommended.

Topics related to bone tissue are now put aside for a while, and the next three chapters introduce ultrasound physics and applications in Medicine.

References

Byrne, D. P., Lacroix, D., Prendergast, P. J. (2011). Simulation of fracture healing in the tibia: mechanoregulation of cell activity using a lattice modeling approach. *Journal of Orthopaedic Research, 29*, 1496-1503.

Carter, D. R., & Beaupré, G. S. (2001). *Skeletal Function and Form: Mechanobiology of Skeletal Development, Aging, and Regeneration (1st edition)*. Cambridge, UK: Cambridge University Press.

Carter, D. R., Beaupré, G. S., Giori, N. J., & Helms, J. A. (1998). Mechanobiology of Skeletal Development. *Clinical Orthopaedics and Related Research, 355S*, S41-S55.

Carter, D. R., Blenman, P. R., & Beaupré, G. S. (1988). Correlations between mechanical stress history and tissue differentiation in initial fracture healing. *Journal of Orthopaedic Research, 6*, 736–748.

Claes, L. E., & Heigele, C. A. (1999). Magnitudes of local stress and strain along bony surfaces predict the course and type of fracture healing. *Journal of Biomechanics, 32*, 255-266.

Claes, L., & Willie, B. (2007). The enhancement of bone regeneration by ultrasound. *Progress in Biophysics & Molecular Biology, 93*, 384-398.

Dimitriou, R., Tsiridis, E., & Giannoudis, P. V. (2005). Current concepts of molecular aspects of bone healing. *Injury, 36*, 1392-1404.

Isaksson, H., Wilson, W., van Donkelaar, C. C., Huiskes, R., & Ito, K. (2006a). Comparison of biophysical stimuli for mechano-regulation of tissue differentiation during fracture healing. *Journal of Biomechanics, 39*, 1507-1516.

Isaksson, H., van Donkelaar, C. C., Huiskes, R., & Ito, K. (2006b). Corroboration of mechanoregulatory algorithms for tissue differentiation during fracture healing: Comparison with in vivo results. *Journal of Orthopaedic Research, 24*, 898-907.

Isaksson, H., van Donkelaar, C. C., Huiskes, R., & Ito, K. (2008). A mechano-regulatory bone-healing model incorporating cell-phenotype specific activity. *Journal of Theoretical Biology, 252*, 230-246.

Hadjiargyrou, M., McLeod, K., Ryaby, J. P., & Rubin, C. (1998). Enhancement of fracture healing by low intensity ultrasound. *Clinical Orthopaedics and Related Research, 355S*, S216-S229.

Kanararis, N. K., & Giannoudis, P. V. (2007). The health economics of the treatment of long-bone non-unions. *Injury, 38*, S77-S84.

Lacroix, D., & Prendergast, P. J. (2002). A mechano-regulation model for tissue differentiation during fracture healing: analysis of gap size and loading. *Journal of Biomechanics, 35*, 1163–1171.

Martin, R. B., Burr, D. B., & Sharkey, N. A. (2010). *Skeletal Tissue Mechanics* (1st edition). New York, NY: Springer-Verlag.

Pauwels, F. (1980). *Biomechanics of the Locomotor Apparatus* (1st edition). Berlin: Springer-Verlag.

Phillips, A. M. (2005). Overview of the fracture healing cascade. *Injury, 36S*, S5-S7.

Prendergast, P. J., Huiskes, R., & Soballe, K. (1997). Biophysical stimuli on cells during tissue differentiation at implant interfaces. *Journal of Biomechanics, 30*, 539–548.

Siska, P. A., Gruen, G. S., & Pape, H. C. (2008). External adjuncts to enhance fracture healing: what is the role of ultrasound? *Injury, 39*, 1095-1105.

Section II - Basics of Ultrasound Physics

Chapter 4

Acoustic Wave Propagation

Abstract

Ultrasound is a mechanical disturbance of a medium, caused by a vibrational source, which promotes a particle motion: a set of compressions and rarefactions. The vibrational motion of particles can be simply modeled as a system of springs and masses, representing a crystal lattice. Many modes of vibration can be observed. Two of them are the longitudinal (disturbances in the same direction of the propagated wave) and the transverse (disturbances perpendicular to the direction of propagation) waves. The radiofrequency (RF) ultrasound signal can be analyzed in the frequency domain by means of the Fourier transform. The shape of the ultrasound beam is determined by wave interferences and the Huygen's principle, i.e., every point localized along a wavefront becomes a point source which emits a spherical wave. The region nearest the face of the transducer is the near field, or the Fresnel zone, and the second region is called far field, or the Fraunhofer zone. When interacting with biological tissues, the acoustic wave can be subject to specular and non-specular reflection, refraction and absorption. Acoustic energy attenuation is caused mainly by scattering and absorption. The most basic equations governing acoustic propagation are the equation of state, the equation of continuity and the equation of motion. The linearized wave equation is a combination of the latter two.

4.1. Introduction

Ultrasound (US) is the mechanical disturbance of a medium (gas, liquid or solid) with frequency above 20 kHz (frequency when the sound is no audible). Nowadays, it plays a key role in Medicine (for example, cardiology, orthopedics, obstetrics and gynecology etc.).

After World War II, the high development in sonar and radar techniques stimulated the use of acoustic sounds in human body. The Dussik brothers (Karl Theodore and Friederich Dussik) were the first to use US for diagnostic purposes, trying to localize brain tumors by through-transmission US attenuation images. Their first paper was published in 1942, with additional conclusions in 1947, after the war.

From this point in time, US has been intensely applied in health sciences, with different imaging properties (linear and three-dimensional arrays, dynamic focusing and apodization, etc.) and several imaging modes (for example, A-mode, B-mode, Doppler, 3D US, etc.). Quantitative ultrasound (the use of ultrasound quantitative parameters for tissue characterization) has also been proposed for several applications, including fracture healing evaluation (subject of this book).

This chapter aims at presenting an overview about acoustic wave propagation. Readers are invited to get detailed information in the bibliographical references.

4.2. Introduction to Ultrasound Physics

It was said that ultrasound (US) is a mechanical disturbance of a medium. This disturbance is caused by a vibrational source, which promotes a similar particle motion in the medium: a set of compression and rarefaction regions (Figure 4.1), in the case of a longitudinal (or compression) wave. The **wavefront** is the name given to the surface joining similar particle positions, which travels at the ultrasound speed. This motion exhibits a sinusoidal pattern, as it can be seen in Figure 4.2. The time between two consecutive cycles is the wave **period** (T), given in seconds, and the number of cycles per unit time is called **frequency** (f), given in Hertz (1 Hz = 1 cycle/s). An important relation between period and frequency is

$$f = 1/T.\qquad(4.1)$$

The distance between two similar points in the wave is called **wavelength** (λ). The maximum value is the wave amplitude. Figure 4.3 shows the relation among three important quantities: the particle displacement, the particle velocity and the excess pressure, which is the change in pressure in a medium (Fish, 1990).

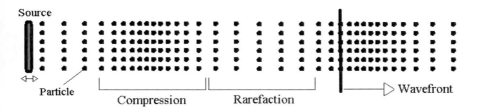

Figure 4.1. Position of particles in a medium after a disturbance caused by the vibrational source. It is possible to observe regions of compressions and rarefactions. This phenomenon occurs with the passage of an ultrasonic longitudinal (or compression) wave. The wavefront is the surface which joins similar particle positions, travelling at the speed of ultrasound.

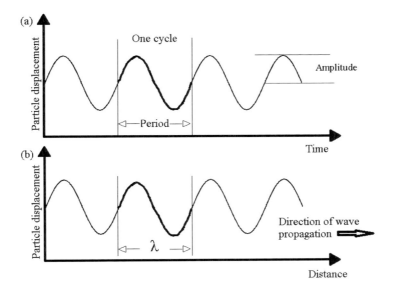

Figure 4.2. A continuous sinusoidal wave. (a) The period is the time between two consecutive cycles, and the amplitude is the maximum value of the wave. (b) The wavelength (λ) is the distance between two similar points.

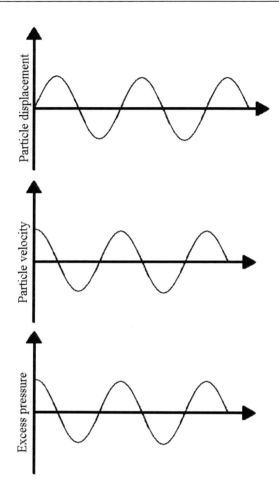

Figure 4.3. Relation among particle displacement, particle velocity and excess pressure.

The vibrational motion of particles in a medium interrogated with US can also be simply modeled as a system of springs and masses (Figure 4.4), representing a crystal lattice. It is easy to understand that many modes of vibration are viable. Two of them are the longitudinal and the transverse waves. **Longitudinal waves** consist in disturbances in the same direction of the propagated wave (also called compression waves), associated with regions of compression and rarefaction. **Transverse waves** are disturbances perpendicular to the direction of propagation, occurring only in solid media (Figure 4.5).

Acoustic Wave Propagation

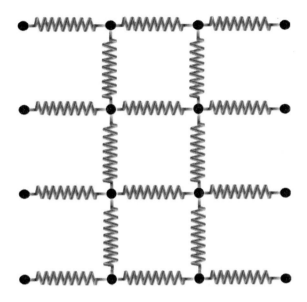

Figure 4.4. A system of springs and masses, for a simple model of a crystal lattice, showing the possibility of many modes of vibration.

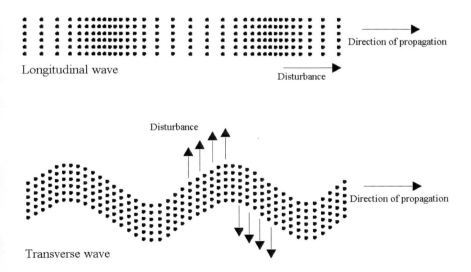

Figure 4.5. Longitudinal (or compression) wave, in which the mechanical disturbance is in the direction of propagation, and the transverse wave, with the disturbance perpendicular to the direction of propagation (occurring in solid media).

The speed of ultrasound propagation (*c*), in m/s, can be calculated using the basic formula

$$c = \sqrt{\frac{E}{\rho}} \qquad (4.2)$$

where *E* is the Young's Modulus (in kg.m^{-1}.s^{-2}), related to the material stiffness, and ρ is the density (in kg/m^3). Therefore it can be concluded that the stiffer the material (increasing *E*) the faster ultrasound propagation is. Some values of *c* in biological tissues are: air (330 m/s), water (1480 m/s), average in soft tissue (1540 m/s) and bone (3500 - 4000 m/s). The speed of sound can be related to frequency, period and wavelength as follows:

$$c = \lambda f \qquad (4.3)$$

and

$$c = \lambda / T. \qquad (4.4)$$

Another important parameter is acoustic impedance (*Z*). At a given frequency, it is the quantity of pressure generated by the vibration of molecules of a medium. Two basic formulae are

$$Z = \frac{P_0}{U_0} \qquad (4.5)$$

and

$$Z = \rho c \qquad (4.6)$$

where P_0 is the excess pressure, and U_0 is the particle velocity; *Z* is given in Rayls (or kg.m^{-2}.s^{-1}).

Ultrasound can be produced in short pulses for many applications. In Medicine, pulsed ultrasound is used for imaging, tissue characterization and therapy. Figure 4.6(a) shows a typical pulse. An ultrasound pulse has a center frequency; however it usually represents the sum of sinusoidal waves with different frequencies. In fact, the frequency components of a signal in time domain can be analyzed using its **frequency spectrum** (signal information in frequency domain). In Figure 4.6(b) it can be identified a maximum peak in 1 MHz, which is the center frequency of the pulse in Figure 4.6(a). Other information from a spectrum is the **bandwidth**, which gives an idea of the pulse frequency distribution. The bandwidth is inversely proportional to the pulse length.

For a frequency spectrum analysis, a simple approach is the calculation of the fast Fourier transform (FFT). Given a signal $x(t)$, the Fourier transform $X(f)$ in frequency domain can be found using the equation:

$$X(f) = \int_{-\infty}^{\infty} x(t) e^{-j2\pi f t} dt . \qquad (4.7)$$

Nevertheless, considering that an ultrasound signal is not an infinite process, we can restrict the limits to a finite time interval, then:

$$X(f,T) = \int_{0}^{T} x(t) e^{-j2\pi f t} dt \qquad (4.8)$$

where the range $(0,T)$ is the time interval considered. The reader may find more information about Fourier transformation and other frequency analysis in more specific books (Bendat and Piersol, 2000; Haykin and Van Veen, 2002).

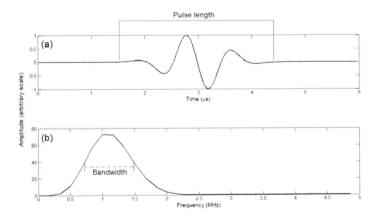

Figure 4.6. (a) A typical 1-MHz ultrasound pulse; (b) the frequency spectrum of the pulse.

4.3. The Ultrasound Beam

An ultrasound beam can have several types of shapes, depending on several factors, like the radius of the transducer (the source of ultrasound waves), frequency and focusing. Two determinants of this shape are wave interference and the Huygen's principle (Fish, 1990).

An interference is the sum of the amplitudes of two waves (constructive interference) or the difference of these amplitudes (destructive interference). This may occur in an ultrasound beam, because the waves are produced out of phase. The **phase** is the time in a cycle of sinusoidally varying quantity (Figure 4.7).

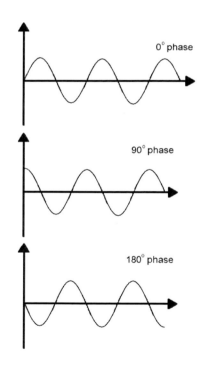

Figure 4.7. Three waves out of phase (0°, 90° and 180° phase).

The **Huygen's principle** (Christian Huygens, 1629 - 1695) is represented in Figure 4.8. It tells us that every point localized along a wavefront becomes a point source which emits a spherical wave (wavelet). Hence it is possible to calculate the wave motion at any point in the ultrasound beam, by adding these wavelets on a wavefront.

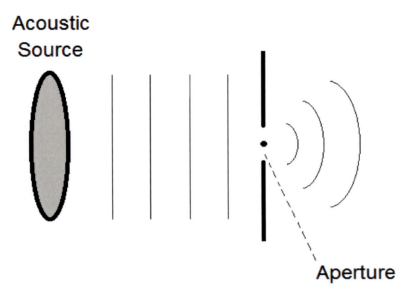

Figure 4.8. The Huygen's principle. The passage of plane waves through an aperture with a point scatter generates spherical waves.

Figure 4.9 shows a common ultrasound beam. The region nearest the face of the ultrasound transducer is the **near field**, or the **Fresnel zone** (Augustine Fresnel, 1788 - 1827). The second region is called **far field**, or the **Fraunhofer zone** (Joseph von Fraunhofer, 1787 - 1826), indicating the point at which the beam begins to diverge. The length of the near field (NF) can be calculated using the equation

$$NF = r^2 / \lambda \tag{4.9}$$

where r is the transducer's radius. The angle of divergence θ can also be found using the following equation

$$\sin\theta = 0.6\lambda / r. \tag{4.10}$$

Another characteristic of these two fields is that intensity varies along the beam axis inside the near field, until it reaches a maximum value (last axial maximum), and then it begins to gradually decrease in the far zone. This intensity variation can be observed when the ultrasound beam is mapped using devices called hydrophones immersed on a water tank (Figure 4.10).

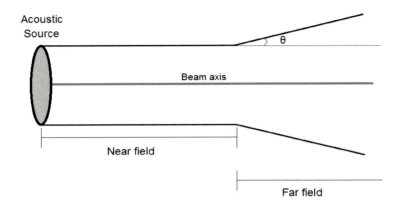

Figure 4.9. The ultrasound beam. The near field (or Fresnel zone) extends until the point where the beam begins to diverge with an angle θ. Beyond that point, the far field (or Fraunhofer zone).

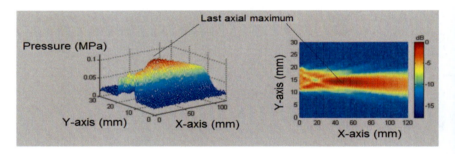

Figure 4.10. An ultrasound beam mapping using hydrophones. It is possible to identify the variation in intensity through the near zone, until reach a maximum (the last axial maxima), which it is related to the beginning of the far zone (Courtesy from Dr. Wagner Coelho - Ultrasound Laboratory, COPPE, Federal University of Rio de Janeiro, Brazil).

4.4. Ultrasound-Tissue Interaction

The acoustic wave interacts with biological tissues in several ways. As the human body presents different types of tissues, for example skin, fat, muscle, vessels and bone, the boundaries (interfaces) between them may cause reflection and refraction. Moreover, the passage of the ultrasonic wave through the medium produces heat (by absorption), promoting an acoustic energy loss.

There are two types of reflection on the boundaries between two media: specular and non-specular reflection. The **specular reflection** is depicted in

Figure 4.11. Let us consider two media: A and B, separated by an interface. When the incident intensity I_i reaches the boundary, it can be reflected to the medium A (reflected intensity I_r) and transmitted to the other medium B (transmitted intensity I_t). The intensity reflection (R_c) and transmission (T_c) coefficients can be obtained, respectively, using the equations (Fish, 1990)

$$R_c = \frac{I_r}{I_i} = \frac{(Z_B - Z_A)^2}{(Z_A + Z_B)^2} \tag{4.11}$$

and

$$T_c = \frac{I_t}{I_i} = \frac{4Z_A Z_B}{(Z_A + Z_B)^2} \tag{4.12}$$

where Z_A and Z_B are the acoustic impedances of medium A and B, respectively. In other words, the reflection and transmission of the acoustic waves are highly dependent on the acoustic impedance difference between the two media. It is also important to consider that, for specular reflection, the angle of incidence equals the angle of reflection (Figure 4.11).

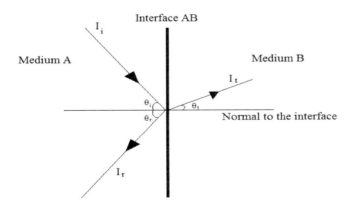

Figure 4.11. Specular reflection and refraction. The incident intensity I_i reaches the interface between media A and B (interface AB), causing reflection (reflected intensity I_r) and transmission (transmitted intensity I_t). In specular reflection, $\theta_i = \theta_r$.

The **non-specular reflection** (also known as scattering) can take place in two situations: (1) when the acoustic wave is incident to a rough boundary; or

(2) when the particles in the medium are small enough compared to the ultrasound wavelength.

When the two media have different speeds of sound, there is a deviation in the path of the incident beam. This phenomenon is called **refraction**. The Snell's law gives the relation between the speed of sound and the angles of incidence and transmission:

$$\frac{\sin\theta_t}{\sin\theta_i} = \frac{c_B}{c_A} \qquad (4.13)$$

where c_A and c_B are the speeds of sound from media A and B, respectively (consider again Figure 4.11).

Absorption is another phenomenon occurring when the wave propagates through a medium, and it results in an acoustic energy loss. It is a simple conversion from mechanical to thermal energy by fluid friction. The absorption is present for a range of frequencies, and it reaches a maximum at the so called relaxation frequency. Biological tissues present different relaxation mechanisms, so for this reason the higher the frequency, the higher the absorption.

The loss in ultrasound intensity is called **attenuation**, and it is caused by five basic mechanisms: (1) reflection; (2) refraction; (3) scattering; (4) absorption; and (5) beam divergence. An attenuation coefficient (α in m^{-1}) can be estimated using the equation (Fish, 1990):

$$\alpha = \frac{\Delta I}{I_i \Delta x} \qquad (4.14)$$

where ΔI is the intensity loss from the passage of I_i through the interface layer with thickness Δx. For a value of α_{db} in dB/m, we use the following relation:

$$\alpha_{db} = 4.3\alpha . \qquad (4.15)$$

To estimate the change of intensity with depth, α can be used in the equation:

$$I = I_0 e^{-\alpha x} \qquad (4.16)$$

where I is the intensity at depth x, and I_0 is the intensity at depth zero (Figure 4.12). The attenuation has a strong dependence on frequency. This dependence can be seen in Figure 4.13. The high-frequency components in the frequency spectrum are more attenuated than the low-frequency region.

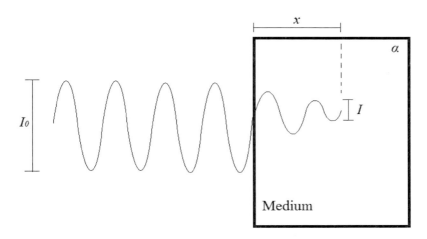

Figure 4.12. Illustration showing the propagation of an incident wave with intensity I_0 through a medium with an attenuation coefficient α. The wave has a decrease in intensity (I) after travelling a depth x.

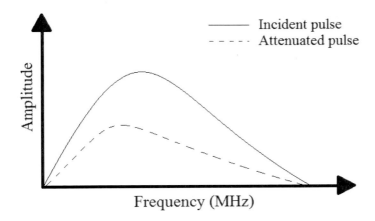

Figure 4.13. Frequency spectrum of an incident pulse and an attenuated pulse. High-frequency components are more attenuated than the low-frequency ones.

4.5. Governing Equations of the Acoustic Propagation Phenomena

This section of the chapter aims at presenting some important equations governing acoustic propagation. For further details, the reader is invited to get information from classical books, such as "Theoretical Acoustics" (Morse and Ingard, 1987) and "Fundamentals of Acoustics" (Kinsler et al., 2000), as well as a more recent book from Cobbold (2007) "Foundations of Biomedical Ultrasound".

First of all, some assumptions are necessary:

- The effects of gravitational forces are neglected;
- The fluid is homogeneous, isotropic and perfectly elastic;
- There are no dissipative effects;
- Acoustic waves are assumed to have relatively small amplitude. Changes in the material density are small compared with its equilibrium value (nonlinear effects are not considered).

It is possible to derive a linearized equation which describes the lossless propagation of acoustic waves in fluids, using three important equations (Kinsler et al., 2000): the equation of state, the equation of continuity, and the equation of motion (Euler's equation).

The **equation of state** relates thermodynamic parameters (pressure and density), and it is written as follows

$$p \approx B_{ad} s \tag{4.17}$$

where p is the excess pressure at any point, B_{ad} is the adiabatic bulk modulus, and s is the condensation at any point. Considering that ρ and ρ_0 are the fluid instantaneous and constant equilibrium densities, respectively, and P is the instantaneous pressure at any point, we have

$$B_{ad} = \rho_0 \left(\frac{\partial P}{\partial \rho} \right)_{\rho_0} \tag{4.18}$$

and

$$s = \frac{\rho - \rho_0}{\rho_0} \qquad (4.19)$$

where $|s| \ll 1$.

The **equation of continuity** is a relation between the particle velocity and the instantaneous density, therefore relating the fluid motion to its compression or rarefaction cycles. The linearized continuity equation is given by

$$\frac{\partial s}{\partial t} + \nabla . \vec{u} \approx 0 \qquad (4.20)$$

where $\vec{u}$ is the particle velocity.

The application of Newton's second law gives the **equation of motion** (Euler's equation), valid for small amplitude acoustic processes:

$$\rho_0 \frac{\partial \vec{u}}{\partial t} \approx -\nabla p. \qquad (4.21)$$

The combination of these three equations yield the **linearized wave equation**:

$$\nabla^2 p = \frac{1}{c_p^2} \frac{\partial^2 p}{\partial t^2} \qquad (4.22)$$

where c_p is the **phase speed** of the wave, given by

$$c_p = \sqrt{\frac{B_{ad}}{\rho_0}}. \qquad (4.23)$$

A quantity known as **velocity potential** (ϕ) exists where $\vec{u} = \nabla \phi$. Considering an inviscid medium, it is possible to obtain ϕ with solutions to the wave equation (Cobbold, 2007, p. 29-31)

$$\nabla^2 \phi - \kappa \rho_0 \frac{\partial^2 \phi}{\partial t^2} = 0 \qquad (4.24)$$

where κ is the adiabatic compressibility given by the equation (for a constant entropy – s')

$$\kappa = \frac{1}{\rho_0} \left.\frac{\partial \rho}{\partial p}\right|_{s'} \qquad .(4.25)$$

Figure 4.14 shows a plane wavefront in Cartesian coordinates (x, y, z). Considering the unit vector $\tilde{k}$, normal to the surface, and vector $\vec{r}$ (from the origin to any point on the wavefront), ϕ can be given by

$$\phi(\vec{r},t) = \phi(c_0 t - \tilde{k}\vec{r}) \qquad (4.26)$$

where c_0 is the small-signal propagation velocity. For a simple harmonic wave, equation (4.26) can be derived in

$$\phi(\vec{r},t) = \phi_0 e^{jk(c_0 t - \tilde{k}\vec{r})} \qquad (4.27)$$

where k is the wavenumber ($k = 2\pi/\lambda$). Using equations (4.24) and (4.26), then it yields

$$\nabla^2 \phi - \frac{1}{c_0^2} \frac{\partial^2 \phi}{\partial t^2} = 0 \qquad (4.28)$$

It can be also demonstrated (Cobbold, 2007, p. 32-34) that the velocity potential for plane, spherical and cylindrical waves are, respectively, given by

$$\phi = \phi_0 \cos(\omega t - kx) \qquad (4.29)$$

$$\phi = \frac{\phi_0}{r} \cos(\omega t - kr) \qquad (4.30)$$

$$\phi = \frac{\phi_0}{\sqrt{r}} \cos(\omega t - kr) \qquad (4.31)$$

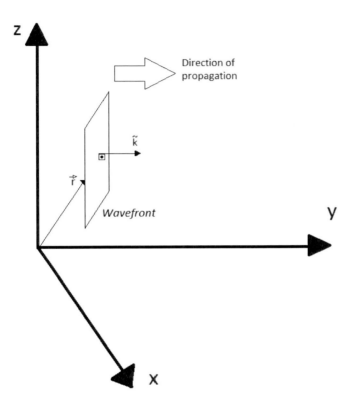

Figure 4.14. A wavefront propagating through a medium (x, y, z). The unit vector $\widetilde{k}$ is normal to the wave surface, and $\vec{r}$ is the position of any point in the wavefront.

For solid media, two velocities will be present: the longitudinal (c_L) and the transverse (c_T) velocities. They can be estimated with the help from the first (λ_l) and the second (μ_l) Lamé constants, which are related to the Young's modulus (E) and the Poisson's ratio (v), for $v \geq 0.5$, in the equations

$$E = 2\mu_l(1+v) \qquad (4.32)$$

and

$$\upsilon = \frac{\lambda_l}{2(\lambda_l + \mu_l)}. \qquad (4.33)$$

Consequently, c_L and c_T can be given by

$$c_L = \sqrt{\frac{\lambda_l + 2\mu_l}{\rho_0}} = \sqrt{\frac{E(1-\upsilon)}{\rho_0(1-2\upsilon)(1+\upsilon)}} \qquad (4.34)$$

and

$$c_T = \sqrt{\frac{\mu_l}{\rho_0}} = \sqrt{\frac{E}{2\rho_0(1+\upsilon)}}. \qquad (4.35)$$

Finally the ratio c_T/c_L can be obtained with

$$\frac{c_T}{c_L} = \sqrt{\frac{0.5-\upsilon}{1-\upsilon}}. \qquad (4.36)$$

For most of the solid media, $c_T/c_L \approx 1/2$.

Conclusion

This chapter introduced the basic aspects of the acoustic wave propagation phenomenon. Ultrasound can be subject to several forms of interaction with biological media, which can be somehow analyzed for tissue characterization. The physical understanding of this process is crucial for researchers from health sciences and biomedical engineering.

Since the aim of this chapter was to give an overview of the physics involved, the reader may find more detailed and comprehensive reading about ultrasound beams and acoustic equations in the books "Theoretical Acoustics" (Morse and Ingard, 1987), "Fundamentals of Acoustics" (Kinsler et al., 2000) and "Foundations of Biomedical Ultrasound" (Cobbold, 2007).

References

Bendat, J. S., & Piersol, A. G. (2000). *Random Data: Analysis and Measurement Procedures* (3rd edition). New York: John Wiley & Sons.

Cobbold, R. S. C. (2007). *Foundations of Biomedical Ultrasound* (1st edition). Oxford: Oxford University Press.

Fish, P. (1990). *Physics and Instrumentation of Diagnostic Medical Ultrasound* (1st edition). West Sussex: John Wiley & Sons.

Haykin, S., & Van Veen, B. (2002). *Signals and Systems* (2nd edition). New York: John Wiley & Sons.

Kinsler, L. E., Frey, A. R., Coppens, A. B., & Sanders, J. V. (2000). *Fundamentals of Acoustics* (4th edition). New York: John Wiley & Sons.

Morse, P. M., & Ingard, K. U. (1987). *Theoretical Acoustics* (1st edition). Princeton: Princeton University Press.

Chapter 5

The Piezoelectric Effect and Acoustic Transducers

Abstract

The devices used in measuring systems by converting one form of energy to another are named transducers. Piezoelectricity is a physical phenomenon in which certain solid materials accumulate electrical charges when submitted to mechanical stress. Acoustic transducers (transmitter or receiver) are used in medical equipment to generate and receive acoustic waves. They are basically composed of a thin plate of piezoelectric material with metallic electrodes deposited on it (the lead zirconate titanate, or PZT, and is the most common ceramic used in Medicine). The piezoelectricity can be created in this material by a process named poling. The piezoelectric active element is cased inside the probe, which is also composed by important items: a coaxial cable, a backing material and a matching layer. The transducer can be developed to generate beam focusing. Some equations for beamforming can be derived for simple, continuous-line and circular piston sources.

5.1. Introduction

Transducers are devices used in measuring systems that convert one form of energy (for example, mechanical, electromagnetic, electrical, chemical, acoustic, thermal) to another. Acoustic transducers are of utmost importance for ultrasonic applications. They are widely used in medical equipments to generate and receive acoustic waves.

Certain solid materials accumulate electrical charges when submitted to mechanical stress. This phenomenon is called **piezoelectricity** (from the Greek "electricity by pressure"), or the **piezoelectric effect**, and it is the basis for the production of ultrasonic waves.

The French brothers Pierre and Jacques Curie (Curie and Curie, 1880) were the first to demonstrate the direct piezoelectric effect (an electrical charge resulting from a mechanical force), in 1880, with crystals like quartz and topaz, but only one year later they considered the inverse piezoelectric effect (a mechanical strain resulting from an applied electrical field) predicted by Lippmann (1881).

This chapter presents the basics of the piezoelectric effect and transducers applications. Some important aspects of acoustic beam formation will also be discussed.

5.2. The Piezoelectric Effect

The piezoelectric effect explains how certain solids change their dimensions when an electric field is applied to them. A simple mathematical approach can be derived for piezoelectricity (Arnau and Soares, 2008). The relationship between the piezoelectric polarization vector (P_p) and the stress to which the piezoelectric material is submitted (T_p) can be written as

$$P_p = d_p T_p \tag{5.1}$$

where d_p is the piezoelectric strain coefficient. For the inverse piezoelectric effect, a strain S_p is produced due to the applied electric field E_p as follows:

$$S_p = d_p E_p \tag{5.2}$$

If we consider the elastic properties of the solid, then we have

$$P_p = d_p C S_p = e_p S_p \tag{5.3}$$

$$T_p = C S_p = C d_p E_p = e_p E_p, \tag{5.4}$$

where C is the elastic constant, and e_p is the piezoelectric stress constant.

The piezoelectric effect leads to an increase of the solid stiffness, because the strain in which the material is subjected generates an elastic stress and polarization (equations 5.3 and 5.4). Considering that ε is the dielectric constant, the internal electric field in this solid will be given by (Arnau and Soares, 2008)

$$E_p = \frac{P_p}{\varepsilon} = \frac{eS}{\varepsilon}. \tag{5.5}$$

Considering that:

$$T = T_e + T_p \tag{5.6}$$

where T_e is the elastic stress, a manipulation of equations (5.3), (5.4) and (5.5) yields

$$T = CS + \frac{e^2}{\varepsilon}S = \left(C + \frac{e^2}{\varepsilon}\right)S = \overline{C}S \tag{5.7}$$

where $\overline{C}$ is the piezoelectrically stiffened constant.

5.3. Acoustic Transducers and Probes

Transducers are devices basically composed of a thin plate of piezoelectric material with metallic electrodes deposited on it (Figure 5.1). The lead zirconate titanate, or PZT, is the most common ceramic used for medical applications. The piezoelectricity is created in this material by a process named poling (a lining up of molecules in a preferred direction).

Acoustic transducers can be used as (Fish, 1990):

- Acoustic receiver: the compression or stretching of the piezoelectric material (caused by an acoustic wave, for example) produces a potential difference, and the electrodes will detect this phenomenon; and

- Acoustic source (transmitter): the application of voltage by electrodes will change dimensions in the piezoelectric material, leading to the production of a mechanical vibration.

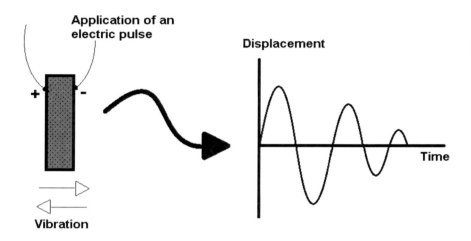

Figure 5.1. A transducer being submitted to a voltage (electric pulse) generates a vibration (displacement) in time.

An important characteristic to be discussed is **resonance**. Any system tends to oscillate at greater amplitude at some frequencies than at others. In this context, each transducer has a resonance frequency in which small forces produce large amplitude oscillations. Consider now the transducer in Figure 5.2, presenting thickness d_t. In addition to wave A, a wave B is formed from the reflection in the second surface of the transducer. The two waves are summed (constructive interference) to generate a greater amplitude wave. There are some conditions to maximize this interference (Fish, 1990), producing waves in phase. Since λ_t and c_t is the wavelength and speed of sound in the transducer material, respectively,

$$d_t = \frac{\lambda_t}{2} \tag{5.8}$$

and the resonance frequency f_r can be found using the expression

$$f_r = \frac{c_t}{\lambda_t} = \frac{c_t}{2d_t}. \quad (5.9)$$

It is important to say that a transducer may have other resonances at integer multiples of f_r, called harmonics.

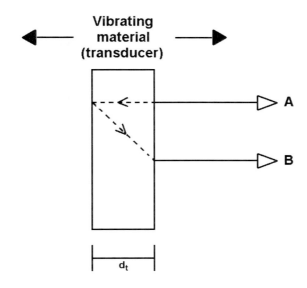

Figure 5.2. A surface of a transducer with thickness d_t producing wave A also produces a wave on the opposite side, which is reflected at the second surface, producing wave B. If A and B are in a phase, a maximum constructive interference will be obtained.

The piezoelectric active element (transducer material) is cased inside the **probe**. The ultrasound probe for a single-element device may present several construction details, but it is usually made of five components: the coaxial cable or connector, the backing, the metal case, the transducer (active element) and the matching layer (Figure 5.3) (San Emeterio and Ramos, 2008). All is constructed inside a **metal case**. The **coaxial cable** makes the electrical connection with the transducer. The **backing** is a high attenuating material, fixed to the back of the transducer, providing electrical shielding (preventing interferences) for acoustic reception and avoiding signals transmission backwards for acoustic emission. Another important item is the **matching layer**, which solves the problem of high acoustic impedance difference between the transducer element and the insonified medium. It is a layer made from a material with the thickness of one-quarter wavelength, and an acoustic impedance between that of tissue and transducer. The ideal impedance of this layer, Z_{layer}, can be estimated using the equation

$$Z_{layer} = \sqrt{Z_t Z_0}, \qquad (5.10)$$

where Z_t and Z_0 are the transducer and tissue impedances, respectively.

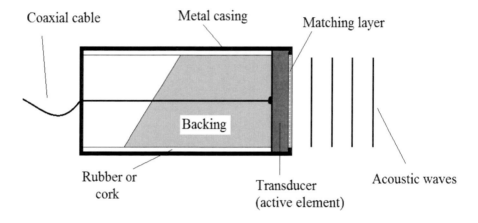

Figure 5.3. A single-element ultrasound probe and its basic elements: a coaxial cable, the metal casing, the backing, the transducer and the matching layer. An acoustic isolator (rubber or cork) is used inside the case.

The backing material is commonly used for imaging probes (pulsed operation), and it is not present for therapeutic purposes (continuous wave). Inasmuch as moisture is not appropriated inside the probe structure, an adequate sealing is very important to avoid undesirable electrical events and any kind of component damaging (Fish, 1990).

The use of **focusing** is essential to obtain narrower beam widths, which is advantageous for some applications. Focusing can be simply accomplished by forming a concavity in the transducer. The degree of focusing will be proportional to the curvature radius. Since there is diffraction spread of the ultrasound beam in the far field, the narrower beam width can only be obtained at the end of the near field and the beginning of the far field. Figure 5.4 shows the variation in beam focusing with different transducer curvature radius.

The focal width W_{focal} can be determined using the equation

$$W_{focal} = \frac{R\lambda}{a} \qquad (5.11)$$

where R is the curvature radius of the transducer.

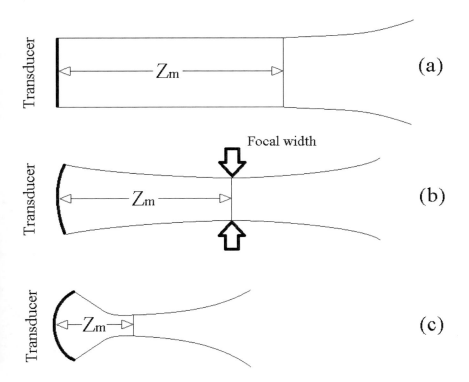

Figure 5.4. Beam shapes from (a) a plane transducer; (b) a weak focusing transducer; and (c) a strong focusing transducer. Z_m is the near zone length.

5.4. Beamforming

It was said in Chapter 4 that an ultrasound beam can have several types of shapes, depending on the radius of the emitter transducer, frequency and focusing, and two aspects are a determinant for its shape: wave interference and the Huygen's principle. The aim here is to give some basic equations to predict field profile for several types of aperture. It is possible to obtain a more complete mathematical approach in acoustic physics books like "Theoretical Acoustics" (Morse and Ingard, 1987), "Fundamentals of Acoustics" (Kinsler et al., 2000), "Diagnostic Ultrasound Imaging" (Szabo, 2004), and "Foundations of Biomedical Ultrasound" (Cobbold, 2007).

A pulsating sphere is considered as the simplest acoustic source. Although it is very difficult to construct, its mathematical approach is important for the idealization of **simple sources**. Some characteristics of a simple source are (Kinsler et al., 2000): (1) it is a closed surface; (2) it vibrates with an arbitrary velocity distribution; and (3) all dimensions are much smaller than the wavelength of the emitted wave.

It can be demonstrated (Kinsler et al, 2000, p. 171-176) that the pressure field of a simple source $\vec{p}(r,t)$, where r is any position in the wavefront, may be written as

$$\vec{p}(r,t) = j\rho_0 c \frac{Qk}{4\pi r} e^{j(\omega t - kr)} \qquad (5.12)$$

where ρ_0 is the constant equilibrium density, c is the speed of sound, k is the wavenumber ($k = 2\pi/\lambda$), r is the position in the wavefront (radius of the spherical beam), ω is the angular frequency ($\omega = 2\pi f$, where f is the temporal frequency), and Q is the complex source strength, given by

$$Q = 4\pi a^2 U_0 \qquad (5.13)$$

where a is the average radius, and U_0 is the speed amplitude. The pressure amplitude P is given by

$$P = \frac{1}{2}\rho_0 c \frac{Q}{\lambda r}, \qquad (5.14)$$

the intensity $I(r)$ is

$$I(r) = \frac{1}{8}\rho_0 c \left(\frac{Q}{\lambda r}\right)^2 \qquad (5.15)$$

and, finally, the power radiated Π can be calculated using the expression

$$\Pi = \frac{\pi}{2} \rho_0 c \left(\frac{Q}{\lambda}\right)^2 \tag{5.16}$$

In practical applications, the ultrasound source is not free of boundaries. A perfect rigid plane boundary is often closed to the emitter, which is called a baffle. The pressure field
$\vec{p}(r,t)$, as seen in Figure 5.5, will be twice that generated by the source alone, because the pressure of the reflected wave on the baffle and that of the incident wave are in phase. This new condition can be observed in the equations

$$\vec{p}(r,t) = j\rho_0 c \frac{Qk}{2\pi r} e^{j(\omega t - kr)}, \tag{5.17}$$

$$I(r) = \frac{1}{2} \rho_0 c \left(\frac{Q}{\lambda r}\right)^2, \tag{5.18}$$

$$\Pi = \pi \rho_0 c \left(\frac{Q}{\lambda}\right)^2 \tag{5.19}$$

respectively, for baffled pressure field, intensity and power radiated.

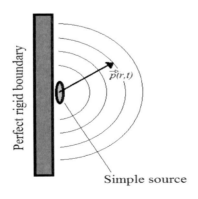

Figure 5.5. A simple source radiating waves close to a perfect rigid plane boundary (baffle).

Another source configuration is the continuous-line source, as shown in Figure 5.5. Equations for the pressure field and the acoustic pressure amplitude in the far field can be written (Kinsler et al., 2000, p. 172-173), respectively,

$$\vec{p}(r,\theta,t) = \frac{1}{2} j\rho_0 c \frac{Qk}{2\pi r} e^{j(\omega t - kr)} \frac{\sin x}{x} \qquad (5.20)$$

$$P(r,\theta) = \frac{1}{2} \rho_0 c \frac{Qk}{2\pi r} H(\theta) \qquad (5.21)$$

where $H(\theta)$ is

$$H(\theta) = \left| \frac{\sin x}{x} \right|, \qquad (5.22)$$

and x is

$$x = \frac{1}{2} kL \sin\theta . \qquad (5.23)$$

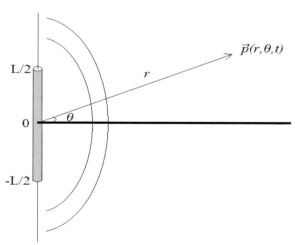

Figure 5.6. A continuous-line source of length L generating a pressure field $\vec{p}(r,\theta,t)$.

The plane circular piston is a common source configuration for several applications, and it is depicted in Figure 5.7. Assuming a flat rigid baffle of infinite extent, the equations for the pressure field in the acoustic axis (z axis) and in the far field (large distances) can be derived (Kinsler et al., 2000, p. 176-179), respectively:

$$\vec{p}(r,0,t) = \rho_0 c U_0 e^{j\omega t}[e^{-jkr} - \exp(-jk\sqrt{r^2 + a^2})] \quad (5.24)$$

$$\vec{p}(r,\theta,t) = j\frac{\rho_0 c}{2} U_0 \frac{a}{r} kae^{j(\omega t - kr)}\left[\frac{2J_1(ka\sin\theta)}{ka\sin\theta}\right] \quad (5.25)$$

where U_0 is the speed amplitude, and $J_1(x)$ is the 1st order Bessel's function.

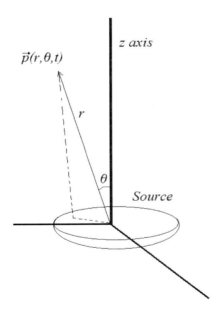

Figure 5.7. A flat circular piston source generating a pressure field $\vec{p}(r,\theta,t)$.

An acoustic beam can exhibit different forms, depending on the source (simple, continuous-line, circular piston). In all of them, a main lobe is always present, containing most of the ultrasound power. Nevertheless, one may observe smaller side lobes outside the main one. Figure 5.8 illustrates (in polar coordinates) a situation where main and side lobes are produced by a transducer. The presence of side lobes is one of the causes of imaging artifacts, which will be discussed later.

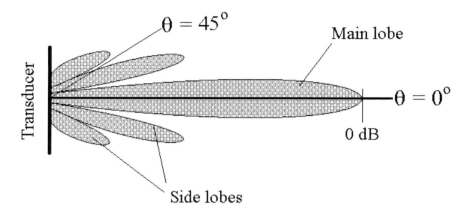

Figure 5.8. A transducer (source) emitting an acoustic beam with main and side lobes (in polar coordinates).

Conclusion

This chapter brought out relevant information about acoustic transducers. These devices are essential for medical ultrasound, because they are the sources and the receivers of the acoustic waves through piezoelectricity.

There are several types of acoustic transducers and probes, according to its applications. The adequate choice of the piezoelectric material, the beamforming pattern, the focusing technique and the probe design play a key role in the generation of desirable diagnostic data, either by imaging or ultrasound parameterization.

The mathematical approach of piezoelectricity and beamforming was also superficially treated in this book. Therefore a more comprehensive reading of the books "Piezoelectric Transducers and Applications" (Arnau, editor, 2008), "Theoretical Acoustics" (Morse and Ingard, 1987), "Fundamentals of Acoustics" (Kinsler et al., 2000) and "Foundations of Biomedical Ultrasound" (Cobbold, 2007) are recommended.

References

Arnau, A., & Soares, D. Jee, W.S.S. (2008). Fundamentals of Piezoelectricity. In A. Arnau (Ed.), *Piezoelectric Transducers and Applications* (2nd edition, pp. 1 – 38). Berlin: Springer-Verlag.

Cobbold, R. S. C. (2007). *Foundations of Biomedical Ultrasound* (1st edition). Oxford: Oxford University Press.

Curie, P., & Curie, J. (1880). Développement, par pression, de l'électricité polaire dans les cristaux hémièdres à faces inclinées. *Comptes Rendus, 91*, 294-295.

Fish, P. (1990). *Physics and Instrumentation of Diagnostic Medical Ultrasound* (1st edition). West Sussex: John Wiley & Sons.

Kinsler, L. E., Frey, A. R., Coppens, A. B., & Sanders, J. V. (2000). *Fundamentals of Acoustics* (4th edition). New York: John Wiley & Sons.

Lippmann, G. (1881). Principe de conservation de l'électricité. *Annales de Physique et de Chimie, 24*, 145-178.

Morse, P. M., & Ingard, K. U. (1987). *Theoretical Acoustics* (1st edition). Princeton: Princeton University Press.

San Emeterio, J. L., & Ramos, A. (2008). Models of Piezoelectric Transducers Used in Broadband Ultrasonic Applications. In A. Arnau (Ed.), *Piezoelectric Transducers and Applications* (2nd edition, pp. 97 – 116). Berlin: Springer-Verlag.

Szabo, T. L. (2004). *Diagnostic Ultrasound Imaging: Inside Out* (1st edition). Burlington: Elsevier Academic Press.

Chapter 6

The Scattering of Ultrasound Waves and Ultrasound Imaging

Abstract

Biological tissues are considered heterogeneous elastic media (regions of different acoustic characteristics), and this diversity in structure gives rise to an intricate scattering phenomenon. This scattering plays an important role on ultrasound imaging (and other ultrasound diagnostic methods). A parameter called frequency-dependent backscatter coefficient can be applied to characterize biological tissues. Although ultrasound imaging is highly operator-dependent, it presents several advantages such as the possibility of soft tissues imaging, the rendering of real-time images, the evidence of no possible harms (non-ionizing), the relatively low-cost and the simplicity to carry out. A first approach of ultrasound imaging is the A-mode, which uses the time of flight of the echo emitted from a transducer to a reflector and back again to the same transducer. The B-mode enables the generation of images putting together a series of A-mode lines. The speckle, a granular texture filling the biological structures (resulting from the interaction of ultrasonic wave and randomly distributed scatterers in the medium), is a very important feature of B-mode images. The Doppler ultrasound imaging makes use of the Doppler effect (the frequency shift that takes place when a propagating wave is reflected by a moving scatterer) to assess the blood flow in body vessels and heart chambers. Other interesting techniques of ultrasound imaging are the scanning acoustic microscopy (using frequencies from 50 MHz to 2 GHz), the ultrasonic computed tomography, and the parametric ultrasound imaging.

6.1. Introduction

Ultrasound applications in medical domain are very challenging. It is not just sending some acoustic waves in a fluid or solid and easily interpreting the echoes from human body. Biological tissues are complex living structures. Changes in metabolism and temperature, cellular development processes, the existence of a disease or a healing event, are factors which may alter the mechanical responses to the passage of ultrasound. Therefore, scientists worldwide continue to investigate techniques to better extract information from backscattered ultrasound signals.

Biological tissues are considered heterogeneous elastic media. This diversity in structure and organization gives rise to an intricate scattering phenomenon. Ultrasound imaging (and other ultrasound diagnostic methods) tries to characterize healthy and pathological conditions, evaluating changes in the acoustic scattering patterns.

The present chapter aims at developing a brief theoretical background about ultrasound scattering from biological tissues, in order to finally discuss some ultrasound imaging methods used for medical diagnosis. More information can also be found in "Theoretical Acoustics" (Morse and Ingard, 1987), "Diagnostic Ultrasound Imaging" (Szabo, 2004), "Foundations of Biomedical Ultrasound" (Cobbold, 2007) and "Ultrasonic Scattering in Biological Tissues" (Shung and Thieme, 1993).

6.2. Wave Scattering from Biological Tissues

A very useful terminology in medical acoustics is the classification of tissue regions in three groups: homogeneous, inhomogeneous and heterogeneous tissue (Szabo, 2004), as represented in Figure 6.1. A **homogeneous tissue** region presents the same parameter value at every spatial point. In the imaging process, it would be a region composed of only one color, or one gray level. An **inhomogeneous tissue** is more applicable for medical purposes, being regions of small parameter values fluctuations about a mean value (even the most regular tissues in the human body present some degree of diversity in structure and organization). Finally, **heterogeneous tissues** have regions of different acoustic characteristics, which can be highly distinguishable from other structures.

The Scattering of Ultrasound Waves and Ultrasound Imaging 91

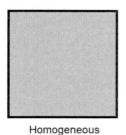 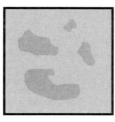 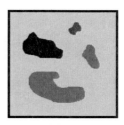

Homogeneous tissue   Inhomogeneous tissue   Heterogeneous tissue

Figure 6.1. Terminology for tissue structures: homogeneous (same values at every spatial point), inhomogeneous (small fluctuations about a mean value) and heterogeneous (regions with different acoustic characteristics) tissues.

A classification from Greenleaf and Sehgal (1992) divides tissue scattering into five distinct classes:

- Class 0: scattering from a molecular solvent on a length scale of 10^{-10} m. Macromolecular effects are considered (absorption and velocity dispersion). Remembering that the attenuation of ultrasound depends on the scattering and/or absorption during its propagation, it can be said that Class 0 scattering reduces wave energy by means of absorption (there is no scattering; homogeneous tissue).
- Class 1: scattering from a concentration of living cells (25 cells per resolution cell), resulting in speckle (a random interference pattern from ultrasound imaging), and $ka \ll 1$ (k is the wavenumber, and a is the scatterer radius);
- Class 2: scattering from a lower concentration (< one per resolution cell). The scatterers can be distinguishable on a image;
- Class 3: scattering associated with organ boundaries, and $ka \gg 1$;
- Class 4: scattering from tissue in motion, as observed in blood.

It is possible to estimate the magnitude of wave scattering by several ways. For a classical approach (Szabo, 2004; Pereira et al., 2008), consider that the scattered intensity I_s from a spherical scatterer (Figure 6.2), can be calculated using the equation

$$I_s = \frac{W_s}{4\pi r^2} \tag{6.1}$$

where W_s is the scattered power, and r is the sphere radius. W_s is given by

$$W_s = \sigma_t I_i \qquad (6.2)$$

where σ_t is the scattering cross-section, I_i is the incident intensity.

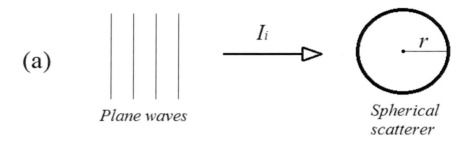

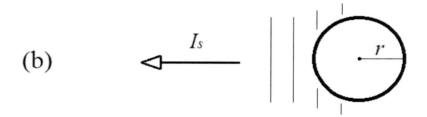

Figure 6.2. (a) Plane waves with intensity I_i are propagating towards the spherical scatterer with radius r (b) generating scattering waves with intensity I_s.

A parameter called frequency-dependent **backscatter coefficient** - $\sigma(f)$ - can be used in several applications, mainly in quantitative ultrasound (QUS), which is a technique aiming at characterizing biological tissues by means of defining parameters related to their acoustical properties. A spectral method is used (for example, the short-time Fourier transform - STFT) and $\sigma(f)$ (in cm.Sr^{-1}) can be calculated with the following equation (Roberjot et al., 1996; Lizzi et al., 1988; Fink and Cardoso, 1984):

$$\sigma(f) = \frac{\langle S_s(f,F)\rangle}{S_p(f,F)} \cdot \frac{1}{(0.63)^2} \cdot \frac{R_p^2 k^2 a^2}{8\pi d\left[1+\left(\dfrac{ka^2}{4F}\right)^2\right]} \quad (6.3)$$

where a is the transducer radius, F is the focal length, R_p is the amplitude reflection coefficient of the reflector plane, $\langle S_s(f,F)\rangle$ is the spatially averaged apparent backscattered power spectrum of the sample (at the focal length), and $S_p(f,F)$ is the reference power spectrum obtained from a plane reflector at the focal length. A Hamming gating function is used to select the region of interest (ROI) from the received ultrasound signal (see Bendat and Piersol, 2000). The factor $1/(0.63)^2$ compensates the application of this procedure.

The Integrated Backscatter Coefficient (IBC) is widely used for biological tissue characterization (Fournier et al., 2001; Meziri et al., 2004; Bridal et al., 2006) and is an integral of the backscattered coefficient given, in decibels:

$$IBC_{dB} = \frac{\int_{f_{min}}^{f_{max}} [\eta(f)]_{dB} df}{f_{max} - f_{min}} \quad (6.4)$$

where $\eta(f) = 10\log_{10}(\sigma(f))$, and $\sigma(f)$ is obtained using (6.3). Several studies have already applied IBC to characterize biological tissues.

6.3. Ultrasound Imaging

According to Szabo (2004), ultrasound imaging (ultrasonography) is the leading imaging modality after X-ray exams. First of all, it presents several advantages: the possibility to image soft tissues like muscle, tendons and organs; it can render real-time images; there is no evidence of possible harm with the use of controlled acoustic intensities; the equipment is relatively inexpensive compared to x-ray and other ionizing diagnostic modalities andsimple to carry out.

Nevertheless, ultrasonography is highly operator-dependent. For an adequate diagnosis, the clinician must be trained and have a certain degree of experience (Wells, 2000). Other negative aspects are the impossibility to image gas-filled body cavities (gastrointestinal tract, lungs), frequency-dependent attenuation (the higher the frequency, the better the image resolution, and the higher the wave attenuation), and for the context of this book, acoustic waves are highly attenuated by bone tissue, hence it is not a gold standard tool for fracture assessment.

Several medical specialties profit from ultrasound imaging techniques, for example (WHO, 1998):

- Orthopedics: soft tissues, bone, muscles, tendons and joints;
- Obstetrics and gynecology: fetal, urine and placental evaluation, examination of the organs of the female pelvis, endovaginal examinations, interventional procedures, breast examinations;
- Cardiology: cardiac anatomy and physiology evaluation;
- Urology: renal anatomy and physiology evaluation;
- Gastroenterology: endoscopic ultrasound of the mediastinal gastrointestinal tract (GIT), liver, gallbladder, pancreas;
- Internal medicine: interventional procedures, echocardiography for diagnosis of visceral and peripheral vessels;
- Surgery: interventional procedures and musculoskeletal examinations.

6.3.1. The A-mode

The first approach of ultrasound imaging was the **A-mode** (*A* means "amplitude"). Generally speaking, it uses the time-of-flight (TOF) of the echo emitted from a transducer to a reflector (scatterer) and back again to the same transducer. Using TOF, the distance d between the transducer and the reflector can be simply estimated using the equation:

$$d = \frac{c.TOF}{2} \tag{6.5}$$

where c is the average US velocity (for soft tissues, $c = 1.540$ m/s). If a medium is composed by two scatterers (Figure 6.3), the distance d between reflectors R_1 and R_2 can be calculated using the expression (Pereira et al., 2008)

$$d = \frac{c}{2}(t_2 - t_1) \qquad (6.6)$$

where t_1 and t_2 are the TOF of echoes from R_1 and R_2, respectively. The received pulse (radiofrequency signal) can be visualized with the help of a cathode ray tube (CRT) display in an oscilloscope.

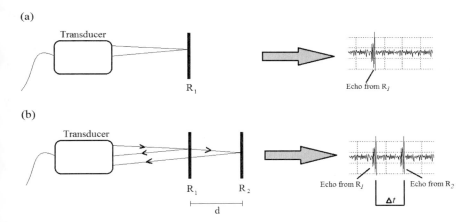

Figure 6.3. A transducer emitting and receiving an acoustic wave in a medium composed of two reflectors (scatterers). (a) The emitted wave travels from the transducer to a reflector R_1, and back again to the transducer, which is registered in the radiofrequency signal (the echo from R1 can be visualized); (b) The emitted wave travels from the transducer to a reflector R_1. Some of the energy is reflected (echo from R1) and some is refracted, being reflected by the second scatterer (echo from R2). Using the time period Δt, it is possible to estimate the distance d.

Figure 6.4 shows a block diagram of a A-scan instrument. Although it is not used anymore in Medicine, the A-mode is extensively used in quantitative ultrasound methods (discussed in details in Chapter 9). The pulse repetition frequency (PRF) generator (or master clock) is responsible for maintaining the synchronicity of all the sections of the equipment. It triggers the pulse generator to excite the transducer, serving also as a time basis for the oscilloscope display. The received signals are sent to an amplitude limiter, and the amplifier increases the amplitude to adequate levels. The time gain compensation (TGC) generator compensates the reduction in signal amplitude as a result of attenuation with propagation depth. The demodulator finds the envelope of the received signal (each burst of the signal transforms into a pulse for each reflector). Finally, the video amplifier prepares the demodulator output to the CRT display (Fish, 1990).

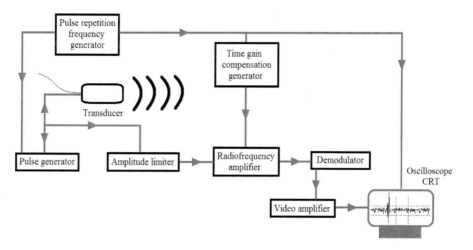

Figure 6.4. A basic block diagram for an A-mode ultrasound instrument.

6.3.2. The B-mode

A series of A-mode lines put next to each other generates an image of a scanning plane called B-mode, where depth is one of the directions. Figure 6.5 shows a sonographic evaluation from a patient with suspected cholecystitis (inflammation of the gallbladder). It is possible to observe the gallbladder boundaries, together with a gallstone inside. The phenomenon called acoustic shadowing can be identified: an artifact in which an intensely echogenic line appears at the surface of structures which block the passage of sound waves. Figure 6.6 is a schematic representation of image formation. A gray-scale image can be observed (for example, with 512 gray levels). In the past, the static B-mode used to produce images from the spatial displacement of a single-element transducer. Nowadays, electronically controlled multi-array probes (composed of several elements cut from one single piezoelectric bar) are available, so the 2D scan is made entirely by circuits (Szabo, 2004; Pereira et al., 2008). These new approaches enabled electronic adjustable focusing and real-time scanning.

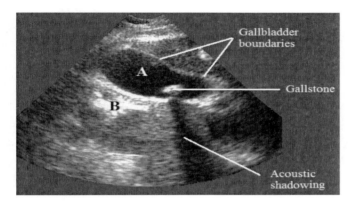

Figure 6.5. Sonographic evaluation of gallbladder from a patient with suspected cholecystitis. It is possible to identify the gallbladder boundaries, together with the gallstone inside, and the phenomenon called acoustic shadowing, produced by the stone. (A) and (B) are, respectively, hypoechogenic and hyperechogenic structures.

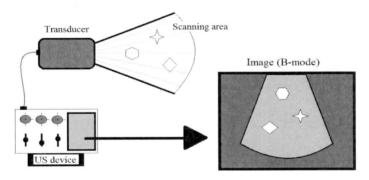

Figure 6.6. Schematic representation of the B-mode imaging principle. Structures can be visualized in gray-scale after an association of A-mode lines inside the scanning area.

A block diagram is shown in Figure 6.7. There are similarities with the A-mode instrument, except for the presence of a probe position sensor that feeds the coordinate generator, and then displays the image in the monitor. The ultrasound image is formed by means of several A-mode lines (signals), which are received by the transducer elements. The signal envelopes are estimated (for example, using a Hilbert transform), and gray-scale values are given according to the echo amplitude (white for maximum echo amplitude, black for echo amplitude zero) (Figure 6.8).

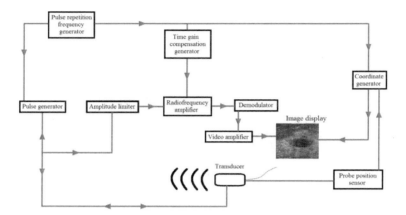

Figure 6.7. A basic block diagram for a B-mode ultrasound instrument.

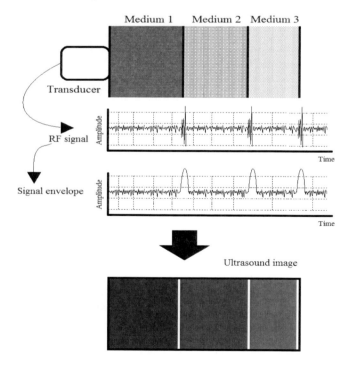

Figure 6.8. Ultrasound image formation. Several A-mode lines (RF signals) are received by the transducer, and an image is produced in gray scale with the help of signal envelopes.

The Scattering of Ultrasound Waves and Ultrasound Imaging

There is an important concept in ultrasound imaging called **resolution**. It is the ability to represent (using an image) structures very close to each other. The **lateral resolution** is defined by the beam focus width (when one scatterer has its diameter smaller then the focus width, the image will be larger than it should) (Figure 6.9). If the distance between two scatterers is greater than or equal to the focus width, they will be imaged separately. The **axial resolution** Δz depends on the pulse length T (Figure 6.10). Consider Δt the interval between the end of the first received US echo and the start of the second one. Then

$$\Delta t = 2\frac{\Delta z}{c} - T \qquad (6.7)$$

where c is the speed of ultrasound. When $\Delta t = 0$, the system axial resolution is calculated using

$$\Delta z = \frac{cT}{2} \qquad (6.8)$$

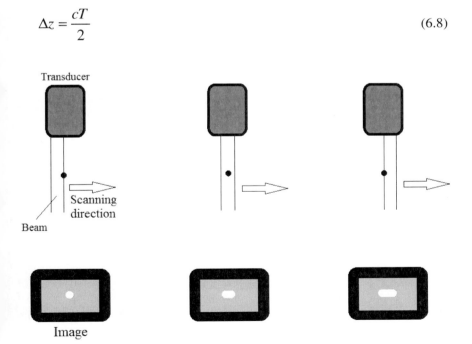

Figure 6.9. An ultrasonic beam is used to image the small black circle, which is smaller than the beam focus width. Therefore, the image will be larger than it should.

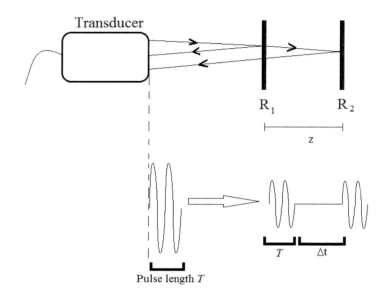

Figure 6.10. Estimating the axial resolution. Two reflectors (R_1 and R_2) can be identified if $\Delta t \neq 0$. The resolution limit is obtained when $\Delta t = 0$.

It is easy to understand that the axial resolution is improved by generating short pulses, although there is loss of energy. Several methods have been developed to compensate for this effect, like pulse compression by wave modulation (Cowe et al., 2007) and coded transmission systems using frequency modulated signals (chirps) (Pedersen et al., 2002).

An important feature in ultrasound images is the so called "**speckle**", which can be visualized in Figure 6.5. It is a granular texture filling the biological structures, resulting from the interaction of ultrasonic wave and randomly distributed scatterers in the medium (Pereira et al., 2008). Investigators worldwide have tried to develop techniques to reduce the effect of "speckle, since it may reduce the image contrast and the ability for detecting subtle tissues changes and boundaries (Dantas and Costa, 2007; Dantas et al., 2005; Chen et al., 2001; Georgiou and Cohen, 1998; Jensen and Leeman, 1994).

Other types of B-mode images are **contrast-media imaging** (use of contrast agents like gas-filled microbubbles encapsulated in a biodegradable shell) (Cobbold, 2007), **tissue harmonic imaging** (using the production of harmonics due to the nonlinearity of sound propagation in tissue) (Michailovich and Adam, 2002), **pulse inversion imaging** (Ma et al., 2005; Burns et al., 2000) and **3D-ultrasound** (Nelson, 2000).

6.3.3. Doppler Imaging

Although Doppler imaging is not used for bone evaluation, it is worth discussing its principles in this chapter, since it is a widely used ultrasound mode in Medicine. The Doppler effect was first described by Johann Christian Doppler in 1842. It is the frequency shift that takes place when a propagating wave is reflected by a moving scatterer. The original emitting frequency (f_o) is increased (if the target is approaching the emitting source) or decreased (if the target is going away from the source) (Evans, 2000). If we consider the same transducer for reception and transmission, it is possible to find the Doppler shift frequency (f_d) with the equation (Evans and McDicken, 2000):

$$f_d = \frac{-2Vf_0 \cos(\theta)}{c} \qquad (6.9)$$

where V is the velocity of the scatterer, and θ is the angle between ultrasound beam and the direction of scatterer motion (Figure 6.11).

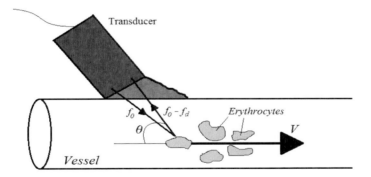

Figure 6.11. The Doppler effect applied to medical ultrasound. A transducer emits a sound wave with frequency f_o which is scattered by a moving erythrocyte with velocity V inside the vessel. The ultrasound beam forms an angle θ between ultrasound beam and the direction of scatterer motion. As the target (erythrocyte) is going away from the source (transducer), the received signal will have a frequency $f_o - f_d$ (f_d is the Doppler shift frequency).

For medical applications, the beam is directed to the blood flow in vessels, and the moving targets are the erythrocytes (blood red cells), and f_d will be proportional to the blood flow velocity (equation 6.9). The use of Doppler ultrasound is concentrated in the assessment of blood flow in body vessels and heart chambers. The Doppler signal is usually transformed in a color pattern in B-mode imaging, placed inside the vessels and cardiac images (Pereira et al., 2008). Figure 6.12 shows an example of a Doppler image from an apparently healthy 30-years old man.

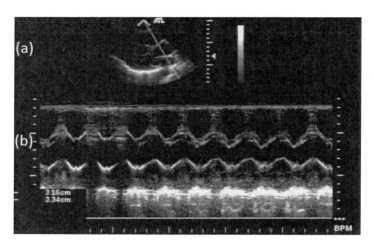

Figure 6.12. A Doppler ultrasound exam from a 30-years old man without previous history of cardiac disorders. The blood flow (a) can be assessed from the cardiac zone showed in (a).

6.3.4. Scanning Acoustic Microscopy (SAM)

The **Scanning Acoustic Microscopy**, or SAM, is an imaging method recently proposed for tissue investigation (using frequencies from 50 MHz to 2 GHz). It is able to extract information of nano- and microscale elasticity of biological media. One of the first instruments was developed by Sherar et al. (1987), using a 100 MHz backscatter microscope to scan a 30-μm thick sample with lateral resolution 17.5 μm. Many studies have been made for applications on ophthalmology, dermatology, and intravascular imaging. Some examples are the evaluation of the anterior portion of the eye with a 50-MHz transducer (Foster et al., 1993; Pavlin et al., 1990) and imaging of skin thickness with frequencies up to 100 MHz (Knapik et al., 2000). Regarding bone tissue assessment, it has been widely used using a pulse-echo configuration for the measurement of acoustic impedance, surface acoustic wave velocities and compressional and shear waves velocities in thin sections (Raum, 2011).

Figure 6.13 shows a representation of a SAM device. The transducer is attached to a spherical lens to focus the acoustic beam. The specimen is placed on a specular reflector, and pulse-echo measurements can be made. In Figure 6.14, SAM images can be seen from a study of Saïed et al. (2008), which aimed at assessing tissue acoustic impedance and microstructure of cortical bone of human radii.

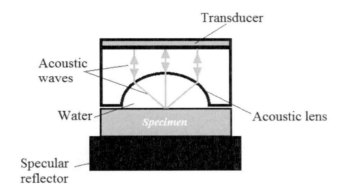

Figure 6.13. A representation of a SAM device. The high-frequency transducer is attached to a spherical lens to focus the acoustic beam. The specimen is placed on a specular reflector, and pulse-echo measurements can be performed.

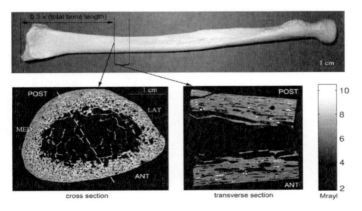

Figure 6.14. A human radius and scanning acoustic microscopy (SAM) images at 50 MHz (Reprinted from Bone, vol. 43, n. 1, Amena Saïed, Kay Raum, Ingrid Leguerney, Pascal Laugier, Spatial distribution of anisotropic acoustic impedance assessed by time-resolved 50-MHz scanning acoustic microscopy and its relation to porosity in human cortical bone, p. 188, Copyright (2008) with permission from Elsevier).

6.3.5. Ultrasonic Computed Tomography (UCT)

The **Ultrasonic Computed Tomography** (UCT) reconstructs the geometry of an object using the spatial distribution of acoustical parameters from backscattered ultrasonic signals. According to Lasaygues et al. (2011), three basic operating modes can be found nowadays, as shown in Figure 6.15:

- A single transmitter/receiver in the reflection mode;
- Several transmitters and receivers in the diffraction mode;
- A pair of transducers (the receiver in the transmission mode), which are translated and rotated around the sample.

Figure 6.16 is an example of a 3D ultrasonic computed tomography from a human fibula (longitudinal length of 2 cm).

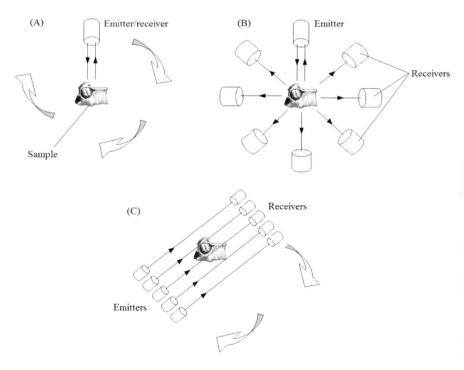

Figure 6.15. UCT operating modes: (A) reflection mode; (B) diffraction mode; and (C) transmission mode.

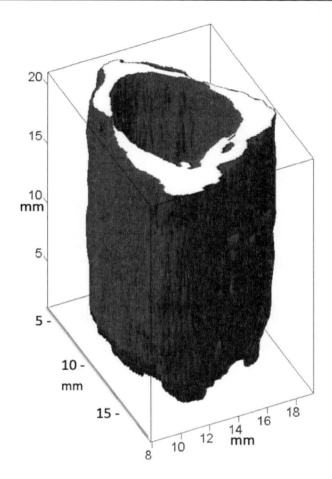

Figure 6.16. Ultrasonic computed tomography (255 x 255 pixels) of a fibula (longitudinal length of 2 cm) from a 10-years old girl (after a surgical procedure). Operating mode: diffraction. Transducer frequency: 2.25 MHz (Courtesy from Dr. Philippe Lasaygues - CNRS - Laboratory of Mechanics and Acoustics - Aix-Marseille University - France).

6.3.6. Parametric Ultrasound Imaging

This method of imaging body structures comes from **Quantitative Ultrasound** (QUS) measurement techniques, and is conceptually simple. QUS parameters (speed of sound, attenuation and backscatter coefficient etc.) can be estimated using backscattered/refracted waves from various spatial points on a sample in order to generate an image. Although QUS has as an important limitation the difficulty in accessing deep skeletal sites (surrounded by soft tissues), some clinical advances have been made. For example the QUS scanner developed by German researcher Reinhard Barkmann and colleagues (Barkmann et al., 2008, 2010). Figure 6.17 shows an example of parametric imaging (using the broadband ultrasonic attenuation, or BUA - more details in Chapter 9) of the calcaneus, compared to an image of magnetic resonance (Chappard et al., 2000). Another example is given in Figure 6.18, where a parametric image of a trabecular bone sample is presented by Karjailanen et al. (2009), measuring the apparent integrated backscatter (AIB) coefficient, a QUS parameter, at 5 MHz.

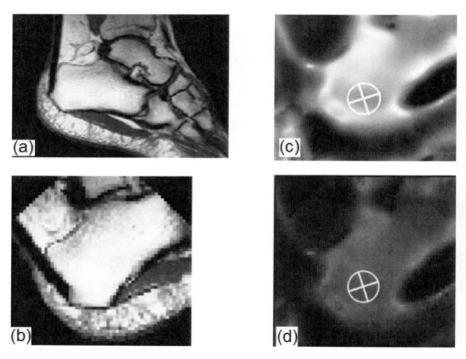

Figure 6.17. Example of the application of parametric ultrasound imaging, using the broadband ultrasonic attenuation (BUA): (a) medial sagittal magnetic resonance (MR) image of a foot; (b) a sub-image after image processing; (c) a BUA image from (b); and (d) a superimposition of BUA and MR images (Reprinted from Journal of Clinical Densitometry, vol. 3, n. 2, Christine Chappard, Estelle Camus, Françoise Lefebvre, Geneviève Guillot, Jacques Bittoun, Geneviève Berger, Pascal Laugier, Evaluation of error bounds on calcaneal speed of sound caused by surrounding soft tissue, p. 124, Copyright (2000) with permission from Humana Press Inc.).

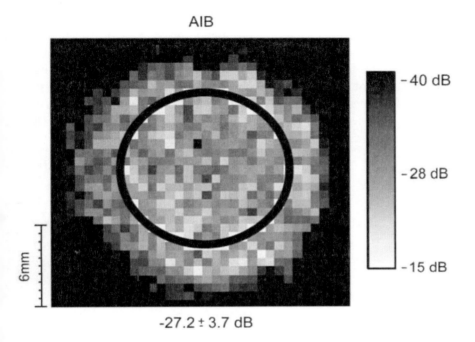

Figure 6.18. Parametric image of a trabecular bone sample, using the apparent integrated backscatter (AIB) at 5 MHz (Reprinted from Ultrasound in Medicine & Biology, vol. 35, n. 8, Janne Karjailanen, Juha Töyras, Ossi Riekkinen, Mikko Hakulinen, Jukka Jurvelin, Ultrasound backscatter imaging provides frequency-dependent information on structure, composition and mechanical properties of human trabecular bone, p. 1378, Copyright (2009) with permission from Elsevier).

Conclusion

Ultrasound scattering is the most important physical interaction between the emitted wave and the medium (biological tissues) for medical imaging. This chapter presented some aspects of this phenomenon, which are essential to understanding how the ultrasound modes like A-mode, B-mode, tomography, acoustic microscopy etc., are generated.

Bone tissue can be considered as an anisotropic material (Chapter 2). The intricate network of trabeculae gives rise to a complex scattering pattern, creating great challenges for researchers. As reflection and transmission of the acoustic waves are highly dependent on the acoustic impedance difference between two media, the interface bone-soft tissue is responsible to a high degree of energy reflection, which generally produces an acoustic shadowing after the cortical boundary in ultrasound imaging. Consequently, the assessment of the body structure is compromised.

With regard to bone fractures, ultrasound medical imaging is not a diagnostic tool of choice in clinical daily practice, notwithstanding some works have demonstrated significant applications, for example, for superficial fractures (mandible, frontal bone etc.) and in bedside emergency rooms. These approaches will be discussed in Chapter 8.

References

Barkmann, R., Dencks, S., Laugier, P., Padilla, F., Brixen, K., Ryg, J., Seekamp, A., Mahlke, L. Bremer, A., Heller, M., & Glüer, C. C. (2010). Femur ultrasound (FemUS) - first clinical results on hip fracture discrimination and estimation of femoral BMD. *Osteoporosis International, 21*, 969-976.

Barkmann, R., Laugier, P., Moser, U., Dencks, S., Klausner, M., Padilla, F., Haïat, G., & Glüer, C. C. (2008). A device for in vivo measurements of quantitative ultrasound variables at the human proximal femur. *IEEE Transactions on Ultrasonics, Ferroeletrics, and Frequency Control, 55*, 1197-1204.

Bendat, J. S., & Piersol, A. G. (2000). *Random Data: Analysis and Measurement Procedures* (3rd edition). New York: John Wiley & Sons.

Bridal, S. L., Fournier, C., Coron, A., Leguerney, I., & Laugier, P. (2006). Ultrasonic backscatter and attenuation (11-27 MHz) variation with collagen fiber distribution in ex vivo human dermis. *Ultrasonic Imaging, 28*, 23-40.

Chappard, C., Camus, E., Lefebvre, F., Guillot, G., Bittoun, J., Berger, G., & Laugier, P. (2000). Evaluation of error bounds on calcaneal speed of sound caused by surrounding soft tissue. *Journal of Clinical Densitometry, 3*, 121-131.

Chen, C. M., Lu, H. H. S., Han, K. C. (2001). A textural approach based on Gabor functions for texture edge detection in ultrasound images. *Ultrasound in Medicine & Biology, 27*, 515-534.

Cobbold, R. S. C. (2007). *Foundations of Biomedical Ultrasound* (1st edition). Oxford: Oxford University Press.

Cowe, J., Gittins, J., & Evans, D. H. (2007). Coded excitation in TCD ultrasound systems to improve axial resolution. *Ultrasound in Medicine & Biology, 33*, 1296-1308.

Dantas, R. G., & Costa, E. T. (2007). Ultrasound speckle reduction using modified Gabor filters. *IEEE Transactions on Ultrasonics, Ferroelectrics, and Frequency Control, 54*, 530-538.

Dantas, R. G., Costa, E. T., & Leeman, S. (2005). Ultrasound speckle and equivalent scatterers, *Ultrasonics, 43*, 405-420.

Evans, D. H. (2000). Doppler signal analysis. *Ultrasound in Medicine & Biology, 26*, S13-S15.

Evans, D. H., & McDicken, W. N. (2000). *Doppler Ultrasound: Physics, Instrumentation and Signal Processing*. Chichester: Wiley.

Fink, M., & Cardoso, J. F. (1984). Diffraction effects in pulse echo measurement. *IEEE Transactions on Sonics and Ultrasonics, SU-31*, 313-329.

Fish, P. (1990). *Physics and Instrumentation of Diagnostic Medical Ultrasound* (1st edition). West Sussex: John Wiley & Sons.

Foster, F. S., Pavlin, C. J., Lockwood, G. R., Harasiewicz, K. A., Berube, L. R., Rauth, A. M. (1993). Principles and applications of ultrasound backscatter microscopy. *IEEE Transactions on Ultrasonics, Ferroelectrics and Frequency Control, 40*, 608-617.

Fournier, C., Bridal, S. L., Berger, G., & Laugier, P. (2001). Reproducibility of skin characterization with backscattered spectra (12–25 MHz) in healthy subjects. *Ultrasound in Medicine & Biology, 27*, 603-610.

Georgiou, G., & Cohen, F. S. (1998). Statistical characterization of diffuse scattering in ultrasound images. *IEEE Transactions on Ultrasonics, Ferroelectrics, and Frequency Control, 45*, 57-64.

Greenleaf, J. F., & Sehgal, C. M. (1992). *Biologic System Evaluation with Ultrasound*. New York: Springer-Verlag.

Hube, R., Mayr, H., Hein, W., & Raum, K. (2006). Prediction of biomechanical stability after callus distraction by high resolution scanning acoustic microscopy. *Ultrasound in Medicine & Biology, 32*, 1913-1921.

Jensen, J. A., & Leeman, S. (1994). Nonparametric estimation of ultrasound pulses. *IEEE Transactions on Biomedical Engineering, 41*, 929-936.

Kinsler, L. E., Frey, A. R., Coppens, A. B., & Sanders, J. V. (2000). *Fundamentals of Acoustics* (4th edition). New York: John Wiley & Sons.

Knapik, D. A., Starkoski, B., Pavlin, C. J., & Foster, F. S. (2000). A 100-200 MHz ultrasound biomicroscope. *IEEE Transactions on Ultrasonics, Ferroelectrics and Frequency Control, 47*, 1540-1549.

Lasaygues, P., Guillermin, R., & Lefebvre, J-P (2011). Ultrasonic Computed Tomography. In: P. Laugier, & G. Haïat (Eds.), *Bone Quantitative Ultrasound* (1st edition, pp. 441-459). New York, NY: Springer.

Lizzi, F. L., King, D. L., & Rorke, M. C. (1988). Comparison of theoretical scattering results and ultrasonic data from clinical liver examinations. *Ultrasound in Medicine & Biology, 14*, 377-385.

Ma, Q., Ma, Y., Gong, X., & Zhang, D. (2005). Improvement of tissue harmonic imaging using the pulse-inversion technique. *Ultrasound in Medicine & Biology, 31*, 889-894.

Meziri, M., Pereira, W. C. A., Abdelwahab, A., Degott, C., & Laugier, P. (2004). In vitro chronic hepatic disease characterization with a multiparametric ultrasonic approach. *Ultrasonics, 43*, 305-313.

Michailovich, O., & Adam, D. (2002). A high-resolution technique for ultrasound harmonic imaging using sparse representations in Gabor frames. *IEEE Transactions on Medical Imaging, 21*, 1490-1503.

Morse, P. M., & Ingard, K. U. (1987). *Theoretical Acoustics* (1st edition). Princeton: Princeton University Press.

Nelson, T. R. (2000). Three-dimensional imaging. *Ultrasound in Medicine & Biology, 26*, S35-S38.

Pavlin, C. J., Sherar, M. D., & Foster, F. S. (1990). Subsurface ultrasound microscopic imaging of the intact eye. *Ophthalmology, 97*, 244-250.

Pedersen, M. H., Misaridis, T. X., & Jensen, J. A. (2002). Clinical comparison of pulse and chirp excitation. *2002 IEEE Ultrasonics Symposium*, 1673-1676.

Pereira, W. C. A., Machado, C. B., Negreira, C. A., & Canetti, R. (2008). Ultrasonic Techniques for Medical Imaging and Tissue Characterization. In: A. Arnau (Ed.), *Piezoelectric Transducers and Applications* (2nd edition, pp. 433 - 465). Berlin: Springer-Verlag.

Raum, K. (2011). Microscopic Elastic Properties. In: P. Laugier, & G. Haïat (Eds.), *Bone Quantitative Ultrasound* (1st edition, pp. 409-440). New York, NY: Springer.

Roberjot, V., Bridal, S. L., Laugier, P., & Berger, G. (1996). Absolute backscatter coefficient over a wide range of frequencies in a tissue mimicking phantom containing two populations of scatterers. *IEEE Transactions on Ultrasonics, Ferroelectrics and Frequency Control, 43*, 970-978.

Sherar, M. D., Noss, M. B., & Foster, F. S. (1987). Ultrasound scatter microscopy images the internal structure of livin tumour spheroids. *Nature, 330*, 493-495.

Shung, K. K., & Thieme, G. A. (1993). *Ultrasonic Scattering in Biological Tissues* (1st edition). Boca Raton: CRC Press.

Szabo, T. L. (2004). *Diagnostic Ultrasound Imaging: Inside Out* (1st edition). Burlington: Elsevier Academic Press.

Van Buskirk, W. C., & Ashman R. B. (1981). The elastic moduli of bone. In: S.C. Cowin (Ed.), *Mechanical Properties of Bone AMD, 45*, pp. 131–143.New York, NY: American Society of Mechanical Engineers.

Wells, P. N. T. (2000). Current status and future technical advances of ultrasonic imaging. *IEEE Engineering in Medicine and Biology, 19*, 14-20.

World Health Organization (1998). *Training in Diagnostic Ultrasound: Essentials, Principles and Standards: Report of a WHO Study Group.* Geneva: WHO.

Chapter 7

Ultrasound Propagation in Bones

Abstract

Bone is considered (macroscopically and microscopically) a highly heterogeneous poroelastic solid. Thus, in order to explain the acoustic wave propagation in this tissue, it is necessary to develop complex mathematical models for its mechanical responses. The knowledge of how ultrasound propagates in solids is crucial to understanding how ultrasound propagates in the bone. Mathematical derivations can be done to achieve the Christoffel equation for uniform plane waves in isotropic and anisotropic media. Some models have been proposed to explain the acoustic propagation in trabecular and cortical bone. The Biot's poromechanical model describes the acoustic propagation in a porous medium saturated by a compressible viscous fluid (inhomogeneous medium), and it is possible to separate the effects of the solid bony frame and the pores filled with marrow (as observed in trabecular bone). Other models for trabecular bone are the Faran cylinder model and the estimation of the frequency-dependent backscattering coefficient. The guided waves technique, a non-destructive testing (NDT) method extensively used for the inspection of plates and hollow pipes, has been recently explored for the characterization of cortical bone and fracture healing process.

7.1. Introduction

The understanding of how ultrasound propagates in bone tissue depends on the knowledge of how ultrasound propagates in solids. Structural rigidity and resistance to changes of shape or volume characterizes a solid (a state of matter), in which the atoms are regularly (crystals, metals, water ice) or irregularly (common glass) bound to each other. In this context, we discussed in Chapter 2 the basics of solid mechanics: the most important mechanical concepts, strength and stiffness, which can be studied from tension, compression, torsion, bending, and shear mechanical tests.

A homogeneous solid can respond to an applied stress, according to three physical models: elasticity (the material returns to its initial form when the applied stress is removed); viscoelasticity (the material behaves elastically, but also presents damping) and plasticity (when the stress overcomes the yield stress, the material behaves plastically, i.e., it does not return to its previous state). However, bone is a highly heterogeneous poroelastic solid (macro and microscopically), hence it is necessary to develop more complex mathematical models for its mechanical responses.

The present chapter aims at presenting a theoretical framework about the propagation of acoustic waves in bones. First of all, some equations governing the acoustic wave in solids will be presented. Afterwards some theories about wave propagation in bones, both cortical (guided waves) and trabecular (Biot's theory) will be discussed.

7.2. Acoustic Wave Propagation in Solid Media

Here a brief theoretical background about the acoustic wave propagation in solid media will be presented. More details can be obtained in important books, such as, "Acoustic Fields and Waves in Solids" (Auld, 1973), "Theoretical Acoustics" (Morse and Ingard, 1987) and "Foundations of Biomedical Ultrasound" (Cobbold, 2007).

Considering the strain field $\vec{S}(\vec{r},t)$ in an acoustically vibrating body, the stress-displacement equation can be given by (Auld, 1973)

$$\vec{S}(\vec{r},t) = \nabla_s \vec{u}(\vec{r},t), \qquad (7.1)$$

where $\vec{u}(\vec{r},t)$ represents the particle displacement field, and ∇s is the symmetric gradient operator, presenting the matrix representation

$$\nabla_s \to \nabla_{Ij} = \begin{bmatrix} \frac{\partial}{\partial x} & 0 & 0 \\ 0 & \frac{\partial}{\partial y} & 0 \\ 0 & 0 & \frac{\partial}{\partial z} \\ 0 & \frac{\partial}{\partial z} & \frac{\partial}{\partial y} \\ \frac{\partial}{\partial z} & 0 & \frac{\partial}{\partial x} \\ \frac{\partial}{\partial y} & \frac{\partial}{\partial x} & 0 \end{bmatrix}. \quad (7.2)$$

The translational equation of motion gives the elastic restoring forces $\vec{T}$ in a freely vibrating medium, and it can be written as

$$\nabla \cdot \vec{T} = \rho \frac{\partial^2 \vec{u}}{\partial t^2} - \vec{F}, \quad (7.3)$$

where ρ is the equilibrium density, and $\vec{F}$ is the applied vector force ($\vec{F} = 0$ for a freely vibrating medium).

A link between the elastic restoring forces and the material deformation must be made. According to the Hook's law, the strain is linearly proportional to the stress, and vice-versa (see Chapter 2). A general linear function of all strain components can be mathematically written as (Auld, 1973)

$$T_{xx} = c_{xxxx}S_{xx} + c_{xxxy}S_{xy} + c_{xxxz}S_{xz} + c_{xxyx}S_{yx} + c_{xxyy}S_{yy} + c_{xxyz}S_{yz} \quad (7.4)$$
$$+ c_{xxzx}S_{zx} + c_{xxzy}S_{zy} + c_{xxzz}S_{zz}$$

and then

$$T_{ij} = c_{ijkl}S_{kl} \quad (7.5)$$

where $i, j, k, l = x, y, z$, and c_{ijkl} is called elastic stiffness constants.

For a cubic crystal, c' can be represented by

$$[c'] = \begin{bmatrix} c_{11} & c_{12} & c_{12} & 0 & 0 & 0 \\ c_{12} & c_{11} & c_{12} & 0 & 0 & 0 \\ c_{12} & c_{12} & c_{11} & 0 & 0 & 0 \\ 0 & 0 & 0 & c_{44} & 0 & 0 \\ 0 & 0 & 0 & 0 & c_{44} & 0 \\ 0 & 0 & 0 & 0 & 0 & c_{44} \end{bmatrix}. \qquad (7.6)$$

For a practical application, consider a x-polarized shear wave propagating along the y-axis (see Figure 7.1), with a stress and strain field, respectively, given by

$$T_6 = T_{xy} = \sin(\omega t - ky) \qquad (7.7)$$

and

$$S_6 = S_{xy} = \frac{k^2}{2\rho\omega^2}\sin(\omega t - ky), \qquad (7.8)$$

where ω is the angular frequency ($\omega = 2\pi f$) and $k = 2\pi/\lambda$ (λ is the wavelength). These fields must be related using the elastic constitutive equation of the propagation medium, given by

$$\begin{bmatrix} 0 \\ 0 \\ 0 \\ 0 \\ 0 \\ T_6 \end{bmatrix} = \begin{bmatrix} c_{11} & c_{12} & c_{12} & 0 & 0 & 0 \\ c_{12} & c_{11} & c_{12} & 0 & 0 & 0 \\ c_{12} & c_{12} & c_{11} & 0 & 0 & 0 \\ 0 & 0 & 0 & c_{44} & 0 & 0 \\ 0 & 0 & 0 & 0 & c_{44} & 0 \\ 0 & 0 & 0 & 0 & 0 & c_{44} \end{bmatrix} \cdot \begin{bmatrix} 0 \\ 0 \\ 0 \\ 0 \\ 0 \\ S_6 \end{bmatrix} \qquad (7.9)$$

or simply

$$T_6 = c_{44}S_6 .\tag{7.10}$$

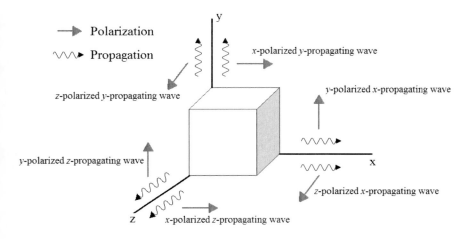

Figure 7.1. Shear waves in a cubic crystal, according to propagation and polarization directions.

The field T_6, S_6 is a valid solution only if

$$c_{44}k^2 = \rho\omega^2 .\tag{7.11}$$

According to Auld (1973), the equation (7.11) is the dispersion relation of the wave, and the phase velocity V_s for this wave can be written as

$$V_s = \frac{\omega}{k} = (c_{44}/\rho)^{\frac{1}{2}}\tag{7.12}$$

Now let us consider a compression wave propagating along the y-axis. The particle displacement and strain field will be, respectively, given by

$$\vec{u} = \hat{y}\cos(\omega t - ky)\tag{7.13}$$

and

$$S_2 = S_{yy} = k\sin(\omega t - ky). \tag{7.14}$$

The stress field can be calculated using (7.14), using the equation

$$\begin{bmatrix} T_1 \\ T_2 \\ T_3 \\ T_4 \\ T_5 \\ T_6 \end{bmatrix} = \begin{bmatrix} c_{11} & c_{12} & c_{12} & 0 & 0 & 0 \\ c_{12} & c_{11} & c_{12} & 0 & 0 & 0 \\ c_{12} & c_{12} & c_{11} & 0 & 0 & 0 \\ 0 & 0 & 0 & c_{44} & 0 & 0 \\ 0 & 0 & 0 & 0 & c_{44} & 0 \\ 0 & 0 & 0 & 0 & 0 & c_{44} \end{bmatrix} \cdot \begin{bmatrix} 0 \\ S_2 \\ 0 \\ 0 \\ 0 \\ 0 \end{bmatrix}. \tag{7.15}$$

then, it yields

$$T_1 = c_{12}S_2 = c_{12}k\sin(\omega t - ky), \tag{7.16}$$

$$T_2 = c_{11}S_2 = c_{11}k\sin(\omega t - ky), \tag{7.17}$$

and

$$T_3 = c_{12}S_2 = c_{12}k\sin(\omega t - ky) \tag{7.18}$$

Since the stress field varies only with y, and $\vec{F} = 0$, the equations

$$\frac{\partial}{\partial y}T_{xy} = -\rho\omega^2 u_x, \tag{7.19}$$

$$\frac{\partial}{\partial y}T_{yy} = -\rho\omega^2 u_y, \tag{7.20}$$

and

$$\frac{\partial}{\partial y}T_{zy}=-\rho\omega^2 u_z \qquad (7.21)$$

represent the equation of motion for a y-propagating free wave. As only $T_2 = T_{yy}$ can enter into (7.19), (7.20) and (7.21) for a wave propagating along y-axis, we have

$$-\rho\omega^2 u_x=0, \qquad (7.22)$$

$$-\rho\omega^2 u_y=\frac{\partial}{\partial y}T_{yy}=-c_{11}k^2\cos(\omega t-ky), \qquad (7.23)$$

and

$$-\rho\omega^2 u_z=0. \qquad (7.24)$$

Substitution of (7.13) for u_y gives us the dispersion relation

$$c_{11}k^2 = \rho\omega^2 \qquad (7.25)$$

which must be satisfied, and the phase velocity V_l (longitudinal wave) is (Auld, 1973)

$$V_l=\frac{\omega}{k}=(c_{11}/\rho)^{\frac{1}{2}}. \qquad (7.26)$$

Since compressional stiffness constants are much higher than shear (transverse) stiffness constants, the compressional waves are faster than shear waves.

7.2.1. Plane Waves in Solids

The following mathematical derivation can be found in a classical book (Auld, 1973). The particle velocity $\vec{v}$ can be given by

$$\vec{v} = \frac{\partial \vec{u}}{\partial t}. \tag{7.27}$$

Then, equation (7.3) becomes

$$\nabla \cdot \vec{T} = \frac{\partial^2 \vec{p}}{\partial t^2} - \vec{F} \tag{7.28}$$

where $\vec{p}$ is the momentum density (in kg/m²s) and it is given by

$$\vec{p} = \rho \vec{v} \tag{7.29}$$

The strain-displacement relation

$$\vec{S} = \nabla_s \vec{u} \tag{7.30}$$

becomes

$$\nabla_s \vec{v} = \frac{\partial \vec{S}}{\partial t}. \tag{7.31}$$

Now (7.28) and (7.31) can be expressed in terms of stress field $\vec{T}$ and particle velocity field $\vec{v}$, considering an lossless acoustic field, using equations

$$\nabla \vec{T} = \rho \frac{\partial \vec{v}}{\partial t} - \vec{F} \tag{7.32}$$

and

$$\nabla_s \vec{v} = \vec{s} : \frac{\partial \vec{T}}{\partial t}. \tag{7.33}$$

By eliminating $\vec{T}$, we have

$$\nabla \cdot \vec{c} : \nabla_s \vec{v} = \rho \frac{\partial^2 \vec{v}}{\partial t^2} - \frac{\partial \vec{F}}{\partial t}, \qquad (7.34)$$

where $\vec{c}$ is the stiffness vector. Then equation (7.34) can be represented in the matrix form

$$\nabla_{iK} c_{KL} \nabla_{Lj} v_j = \rho \frac{\partial^2 v_i}{\partial t^2} - \frac{\partial F_i}{\partial t} \qquad (7.35)$$

where the operator ∇_{iK} is given by

$$\nabla_{iK} = \begin{bmatrix} \dfrac{\partial}{\partial x} & 0 & 0 & 0 & \dfrac{\partial}{\partial z} & \dfrac{\partial}{\partial y} \\ 0 & \dfrac{\partial}{\partial y} & 0 & \dfrac{\partial}{\partial z} & 0 & \dfrac{\partial}{\partial x} \\ 0 & 0 & \dfrac{\partial}{\partial z} & \dfrac{\partial}{\partial y} & \dfrac{\partial}{\partial x} & 0 \end{bmatrix} \qquad (7.36)$$

and ∇_{Lj} has the form (7.2). Considering $\vec{F} = 0$, a uniform plane wave has fields proportional to $e^{i(\omega t - k\hat{l} \cdot r)}$, propagating in the direction $\hat{l}$ given by

$$\hat{l} = \hat{x} l_x + \hat{y} l_y + \hat{z} l_z . \qquad (7.37)$$

The operators ∇_{iK} and ∇_{Lj} can be substituted by matrices $-ik_{iK}$ e $-ik_{Lj}$:

$$-ik_{iK} = -ikl_{iK} \rightarrow -ik \begin{bmatrix} l_x & 0 & 0 & 0 & l_z & l_y \\ 0 & l_y & 0 & l_z & 0 & l_x \\ 0 & 0 & l_z & l_y & l_x & 0 \end{bmatrix} \qquad (7.38)$$

$$-ik_{Lj} = -ikl_{Lj} \rightarrow -ik \begin{bmatrix} l_x & 0 & 0 \\ 0 & l_y & 0 \\ 0 & 0 & l_z \\ 0 & l_z & l_y \\ l_z & 0 & l_x \\ l_y & l_x & 0 \end{bmatrix}.$$ (7.39)

And finally the **Christoffel equation**, applied for uniform plane waves in isotropic or anisotropic media, can be derived from (7.35), for $\vec{F} = 0$:

$$k^2(l_{iK}c_{KL}l_{Lj})v_j = k^2\Gamma_{ij}v_j = \rho\omega^2 v_i ,$$ (7.40)

where Γ_{ij} is the Christoffel matrix:

$$\Gamma_{ij} = l_{iK}c_{KL}l_{Lj} .$$ (7.41)

For the **isotropic case**, the three axes, x, y and z are equivalent to the three planes yz, xz and xy. For this reason, a compressive stress applied along any axis produces the same response. It can be proven (Auld, 1973) that the general stiffness matrix $[c']$ is

$$[c'] = \begin{bmatrix} c_{11} & c_{12} & c_{12} & 0 & 0 & 0 \\ c_{12} & c_{11} & c_{12} & 0 & 0 & 0 \\ c_{12} & c_{12} & c_{11} & 0 & 0 & 0 \\ 0 & 0 & 0 & c_{44} & 0 & 0 \\ 0 & 0 & 0 & 0 & c_{44} & 0 \\ 0 & 0 & 0 & 0 & 0 & c_{44} \end{bmatrix},$$ (7.42)

and the condition for invariance of [c'] with respect to rotation is

$$c_{12} = c_{11} - 2c_{44}. \tag{7.43}$$

Equations (7.42) and (7.43) will show that only two independent elastic constants are present in isotropic media, the Lamé coefficients (see Chapter 4), $\lambda_l = c_{12}$ and $\mu_l = c_{44}$. Using equations (7.42) and (7.43) in the Christoffel matrix (7.41), the Christoffel equation (7.40) reduces to

$$k^2 \begin{bmatrix} c_{44} & 0 & 0 \\ 0 & c_{44} & 0 \\ 0 & 0 & c_{11} \end{bmatrix} \begin{bmatrix} v_x \\ v_y \\ v_z \end{bmatrix} = \rho\omega^2 \begin{bmatrix} v_x \\ v_y \\ v_z \end{bmatrix}. \tag{7.44}$$

which can be split in the following three independent equations:

$$k^2 c_{44} v_x = \rho\omega^2 v_x, \tag{7.45}$$

$$k^2 c_{44} v_y = \rho\omega^2 v_y, \tag{7.46}$$

and

$$k^2 c_{11} v_z = \rho\omega^2 v_z \tag{7.47}$$

For the **anisotropic case**, let us consider the most common type of solid represented by the triclinic system. The transformation matrices for this system are

$$1 \rightarrow \begin{bmatrix} 1 & 0 & 0 \\ 0 & 1 & 0 \\ 0 & 0 & 1 \end{bmatrix} \tag{7.48}$$

and

$$\overline{1} \rightarrow \begin{bmatrix} -1 & 0 & 0 \\ 0 & -1 & 0 \\ 0 & 0 & -1 \end{bmatrix}, \tag{7.49}$$

and when they are substituted in (7.41), the Christoffel equation for triclinic crystals can be derived:

$$k^2 \begin{bmatrix} \alpha & \delta & \varepsilon \\ \delta & \beta & \zeta \\ \varepsilon & \zeta & \gamma \end{bmatrix} \begin{bmatrix} v_x \\ v_y \\ v_z \end{bmatrix} = \rho \omega^2 \begin{bmatrix} v_x \\ v_y \\ v_z \end{bmatrix} \tag{7.50}$$

where the terms in the first matrix are given by

$$\alpha = c_{11}l_x^2 + c_{66}l_y^2 + c_{55}l_z^2 + 2c_{56}l_yl_z + 2c_{15}l_zl_x + 2c_{16}l_xl_y, \tag{7.51}$$

$$\beta = c_{66}l_x^2 + c_{22}l_y^2 + c_{44}l_z^2 + 2c_{24}l_yl_z + 2c_{46}l_zl_x + 2c_{26}l_xl_y, \tag{7.52}$$

$$\gamma = c_{55}l_x^2 + c_{44}l_y^2 + c_{33}l_z^2 + 2c_{34}l_yl_z + 2c_{35}l_zl_x + 2c_{45}l_xl_y, \tag{7.53}$$

$$\delta = c_{16}l_x^2 + c_{26}l_y^2 + c_{45}l_z^2 + (c_{46}+c_{25})l_yl_z + (c_{14}+c_{56})l_zl_x + (c_{12}+c_{66})l_xl_y, \tag{7.54}$$

$$\varepsilon = c_{15}l_x^2 + c_{46}l_y^2 + c_{35}l_z^2 + (c_{45}+c_{36})l_yl_z + (c_{13}+c_{55})l_zl_x + (c_{14}+c_{56})l_xl_y, \tag{7.55}$$

$$\zeta = c_{56}l_x^2 + c_{24}l_y^2 + c_{34}l_z^2 + (c_{44}+c_{23})l_yl_z + (c_{36}+c_{45})l_zl_x + (c_{25}+c_{46})l_xl_y, \tag{7.56}$$

and

$$l_x = k_x/k, \tag{7.57}$$

$$l_y = k_y/k, \tag{7.58}$$

$l_z = k_z/k$ (7.59)

are the cosines in the direction of propagation. With the use of adequate initial conditions, this result can be obtained for other crystal systems.

7.3. The Biot's Poromechanical Model

In 1956, Maurice Anthony Biot, a Belgian physicist, published an important scientific paper providing a description of the acoustic propagation in a porous medium saturated by a compressible viscous fluid, i.e., an inhomogeneous medium (Biot, 1956). His theory was first developed for applications in geophysics. Since trabecular bone can be considered an inhomogeneous medium, theories such as Biot's model has been proposed by many bone researchers (Wilson, 1992; Haire and Langton, 1999; Hosokawa and Otani, 1997, 1998; Fellah et al., 2008; Sebaa et al., 2008).

According to Biot's model, the behavior of the frame and pore fluid has to be treated together, deriving equations of motion for each phase. It can be predicted parameters as acoustic velocity and attenuation in a two-phase medium, depending on ultrasound frequency, elastic properties, permeability, porosity, etc. The theory considers energy loss due to the viscosity of the pore fluid.

The model predicts three wave modes: a compressional wave (called fast longitudinal wave or wave of the first kind), a transverse wave, and another compressional wave called slow wave (or wave of the second kind), using six basic assumptions: (1) ultrasonic wavelength is large if compared to the volume dimensions - scattering effects neglected; (2) mechanical displacements, strain and particle velocity are small enough; (3) adiabatic conditions; (4) the solid frame is isotropic; (5) the fluid phase is continuous; and (6) the stress in the fluid is hydrostatically distributed.

Considering an incident wave perpendicular to the volume surface, it can generate solid ($\vec{u}_s$) and fluid ($\vec{u}_f$) displacements inside trabecular bone, satisfying the equations (Fellah et al., 2008):

$$\tilde{\rho}_{11}(\omega)\frac{\partial^2 \vec{u}_s}{\partial t^2} + \tilde{\rho}_{12}(\omega)\frac{\partial^2 \vec{u}_f}{\partial t^2} = P\vec{\nabla}.(\vec{\nabla}.\vec{u}_s) + Q\vec{\nabla}.(\vec{\nabla}.\vec{u}_f) - N\vec{\nabla} \wedge (\vec{\nabla} \wedge \vec{u}_s) \quad (7.60)$$

$$\tilde{\rho}_{12}(\omega)\frac{\partial^2 \vec{u}_s}{\partial t^2} + \tilde{\rho}_{22}(\omega)\frac{\partial^2 \vec{u}_f}{\partial t^2} = Q\vec{\nabla}.(\vec{\nabla}.\vec{u}_s) + R\vec{\nabla}.(\vec{\nabla}.\vec{u}_f) \; , \qquad (7.61)$$

where $\tilde{\rho}_{mn}$ is the Biot's coefficient, given by

$$\tilde{\rho}_{mn} = \rho_{mn} + (-1)^{m+n}\frac{b}{j\omega} \; , \qquad (7.62)$$

P, Q and R are generalized elastic constants related to the porosity (ϕ), fluid bulk modulus (K_f), solid bulk modulus (K_s) and the bulk modulus of the solid porous frame (K_b); N is the shear modulus of the solid (Sebaa et al., 2008). The mass coefficients ρ_{mn} can be calculated using the relations

$$\rho_{11} + \rho_{12} = (1-\phi)\rho_s \qquad (7.63)$$

and

$$\rho_{12} + \rho_{22} = \phi\rho_f \; . \qquad (7.64)$$

The parameter ρ_{12} is the mass coupling between the solid and fluid phases, and it can be calculated using

$$\rho_{12} = -\phi\rho_f(\alpha - 1) \qquad (7.65)$$

where α is the tortuosity.

It can be defined a dynamic tortuosity $\alpha(\omega)$ (depending on frequency) as follows:

$$\alpha(\omega) = \alpha - \frac{jb\phi}{\omega\rho_f} \; . \qquad (7.66)$$

Substituting $\alpha(\omega)$ in place of α in (7.65), then it can be shown that $\tilde{\rho}_{mn} = \rho_{mn}$. A correction of $\alpha(\omega)$ for a higher frequency range can be deduced to represent viscous exchanges between fluid and solid phase, and it can be given by (Johnson et al., 1987)

$$\alpha(\omega) = \alpha'\left(1 + \frac{\eta\phi}{j\omega\alpha'\rho_f k_0}\sqrt{1 + j\frac{4\alpha'^2 k_0^2 \rho_f \omega}{\eta\Lambda^2\phi^2}}\right) \tag{7.67}$$

where α' is the tortuosity, Λ expresses the viscous characteristic length, η is the fluid viscosity, as shown by Johnson et al. (1987).

A parameter called viscous skin depth thickness can be found using the expression

$$\delta = \sqrt{\frac{2\eta}{\omega\rho_f}} \tag{7.68}$$

which is the region of the fluid in which the the frictional forces at the interface fluid-solid frame disturb the velocity distribution. Therefore the viscous skin δ is very thin near the radius of the pore r, for high frequencies, and only a small volume near the surface of the solid frame concentrates the viscous effects, consequently

$$\frac{\delta}{r} \ll 1 \tag{7.69}$$

For this condition, equation (7.67) can be rewritten as

$$\alpha(\omega) = \alpha'\left(1 + \frac{2}{\Lambda}\sqrt{\frac{\eta}{j\omega\rho_f}}\right). \tag{7.70}$$

Figure 7.2 illustrates an experimental setup for ultrasonic measurements (transmission mode). Considering that the sample with thickness L is interrogated with an incident pressure $p_i(t)$, the transmitted pressure can be given by

$$p_t(x,t) = \int_0^t \widetilde{T}(\tau) p_i\left(t - \tau - \frac{(x-L)}{c_0}\right) d\tau \qquad (7.71)$$

where c_0 is the velocity outside the porous material, and $\widetilde{T}$ is the transmission scattering operator. In the frequency domain, we have the transmission coefficient

$$T(\omega) = \frac{j\omega^2 \rho_f c_0 F_4(\omega)}{(j\omega \rho_f c_0 F_4(\omega))^2 - (j\omega F_3(\omega) - 1)^2}, \qquad (7.72)$$

where $F_3(\omega)$ and $F_4(\omega)$ are given by mathematical expressions which contain the Biot's coefficients. For more details, the reader is invited to read the papers of Fellah et al. (2001, 2008) and Sebaa et al. (2008).

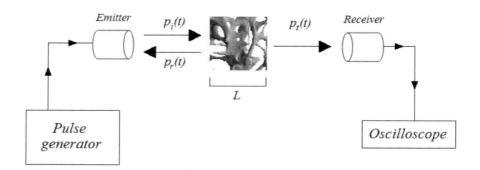

Figure 7.2. A basic ultrasound transmission mode setup for characterization of a trabecular bone sample with thickness L. The emitter produces a wave with incident pressure $p_i(t)$. A reflected pressure $p_r(t)$ and transmitted pressure $p_t(t)$ are generated, the later being captured by an oscilloscope for offline signal processing.

For Pakula et al. (2011, p. 114), the Biot's theory is "an attractive candidate to model ultrasonic wave propagation in cancellous bones because of the two-phase nature of the medium", i.e., it is possible to separate the effects of the solid bony frame and the pores filled with marrow. However, further research is needed. Although significant progress has been made in presenting the potential of Biot's model to predict the waves transmitted through the trabecular bone (Lee and Yoon, 2006; Kaczmarek et al., 2002; Hughes et al., 2003; Pakula et al., 2009), it exhibits mainly two drawbacks: (1)

the great number of input parameters to be used in the equation; (2) it must be considered that ultrasonic wavelength is large if compared to the volume dimensions, then the scattering effects are neglected. Further research is then necessary.

7.4. Scattering Models for Trabecular Bone

The solid trabeculae and the marrow-filled pores present a high impedance mismatch. For this reason, trabecular bone is a strong scattering medium. Figure 7.3 shows a calcaneus sample with the cortical layers removed. The variations in trabeculae orientations are evident.

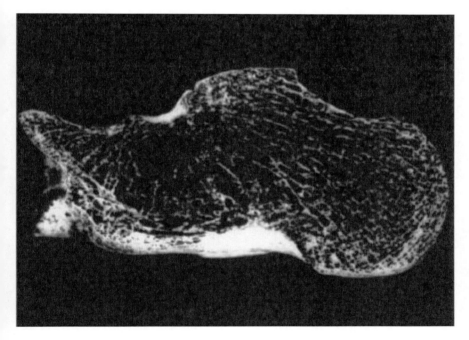

Figure 7.3. A calcaneus sample with the cortical layers removed. It is possible to observe the diversity in trabeculae orientations (Reprinted with permission from The Journal of the Acoustical Society of America, vol. 106, n. 6, Keith Wear, Frequency dependence of ultrasonic backscatter from human trabecular bone: Theory and experiment, p. 3660, Copyright (1999), Acoustic Society of America).

The modeling of this acoustic phenomenon is a hard task, but some progress has been made. For Padilla and Wear (2011), three main problems arise from the analysis of trabecular ultrasonic scattering: (1) the backscattered wave from trabecular bone is a summation of scattered waves from trabeculae at diagnostic frequencies, producing constructive and destructive interferences; (2) bone is a tissue with a high attenuation coefficient, leading to a limited penetration; and (3) the attenuation coefficient is usually measured by ultrasonic transmission experiments, which tends to overestimate this parameter.

Some models of trabecular bone scattering were already proposed. One of them is the **Faran cylinder model** (Faran, 1951), which gives solutions for the scattered pressure from a uniform cylinder:

$$p_s = \sum_{m=0}^{\infty} A_m \cos(m\theta)[J_m(kr) + iN_m(kr)], \qquad (7.73)$$

where θ and r are the cylindrical coordinates, and J_m and N_m are the cylindrical Bessel function of the first and second kind, respectively. A_m are decomposition coefficients and they can be found in Faran (1951).

The **backscattering coefficient** ($\sigma(f)$) can also be used for trabecular bone characterization, modeling it as a medium composed of a fluid and solid inhomogeneities. In one of its formulations (Morse and Ingard, 1987; Padilla et al., 2003), considering no absorption and no multiple scattering effects (called the Born approximation), $\sigma(f)$ can be written as

$$\sigma(f) = \frac{1}{V} \left| \frac{k_f^2}{4\pi} \iiint_V [\gamma_\kappa(\vec{r}_o) - \gamma_\rho(\vec{r}_o)] e^{-i\vec{K}\cdot\vec{r}_o} d\vec{r}_o \right|^2, \qquad (7.74)$$

where V is the scattering volume, $k_f = \omega c_f$ (c_f being the acoustic wave velocity in the fluid), γ_κ and γ_ρ are functions which describe the variations in density and compressibility in bone compared to water, respectively; $\vec{K} = -2k_f \hat{z}$ ($\hat{z}$ is the unit vector in the direction of propagation of the incident wave).

7.5. Guided Waves

Guided waves technique is a non-destructive testing (NDT) method, extensively used for the inspection of plates and hollow pipes, which are considered waveguides (structures which guide waves). These waves arise from acoustic mode conversion between longitudinal and shear waves during the propagation through bounded media (for example, water and metal). In the case of a free plate (homogeneous isotropic elastic plate, traction-free upper and lower surfaces), guided waves are called **plate waves** or **Lamb waves**.

Cortical bone can be considered a waveguide. As seen in Chapter 1, it forms the shaft of long bones and the shell of cancellous bone. Therefore, it is similar to a free plate with soft tissue externally (muscles, for example) and internally (marrow). In this context, several authors have been proposing the application of guided waves for the characterization of bone quality and fracture healing.

One important characteristic of Lamb waves is dispersion (the acoustic velocity within a plate depends on frequency and plate thickness). According to the dispersion pattern from the acoustic propagation through cortical bone, quantitative parameters can be extracted in order to assess clinical conditions like osteoporosis (Moilanen et al., 2008; Talmant et al., 2009) and fractures (Protopappas et al., 2006, 2007; Vavva et al., 2008).

The Rayleigh-Lamb equation describes the dispersion of Lamb waves (Protopappas et al., 2006):

$$\frac{\tan \beta d/2}{\tan \alpha d/2} = \left[-\frac{4\alpha\beta k^2}{(k^2 - \beta^2)^2} \right]^{\pm 1} \qquad (7.75)$$

where d is the plate thickness, k is the wavenumber ($k = \omega/c$), and c is the phase velocity. α and β are given, respectively, by

$$\alpha = \frac{\omega^2}{c_L^2} - k^2 \qquad (7.76)$$

and

$$\beta = \frac{\omega^2}{c_T^2} - k^2 \qquad (7.77)$$

where c_L and c_T are, respectively, the bulk longitudinal and shear velocities.

The propagation of guided waves can generate symmetric (motion symmetric with respect to the midplane of the plate) and asymmetric (motion asymmetric with respect to the midplane of the plate) modes. The exponent ±1 in equation (7.75) will yield solutions for symmetric (+1) and asymmetric (-1) modes. The same equation will also produce the velocity dispersion according to the frequency-thickness ($f \times d$) product (Figure 7.4). Symmetric modes are denoted as S0, S1, S2, etc., and asymmetric modes are denoted as A0, A1, A2, etc. The longitudinal L(0,m), torsional T(0,m) and flexural F(n,m) modes are guided waves forms, where m is the order of the mode, and n is the circumferential order (order of symmetry around the axis).

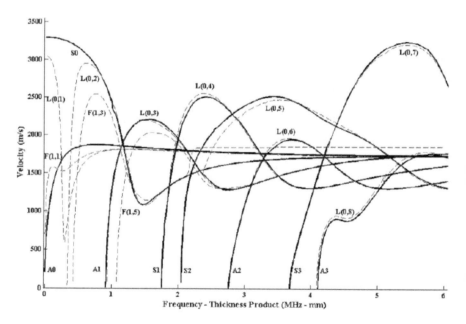

Figure 7.4. Group velocity dispersion curves for symmetric and antisymmetric Lamb modes as a function of the frequency-thickness product. In solid and dashed lines are shown, respectively, the curves for a free plate and a free tube (Reprinted from Ultrasound in Medicine & Biology, vol. 32, n. 5, Vasilios Protopappas, Dimitriou Fotiadis, Konstantinos Malizos, Guided ultrasound wave propagation in intact and healing long bones, p. 695, Copyright (2006) with permission from Elsevier).

7.5.1. The Lateral Wave

The lateral wave (or head wave) is a linear wavefront connecting the refracted to the reflected wavefront. It is generated when an acoustic wave propagating in a fluid reaches the interface fluid-solid, and it presents the same longitudinal velocity from the solid, making an angle θ_c with the interface (Camus et al., 2000; Bossy et al., 2002). The analysis of this wave has been extensively done in the last works about the application of QUS in fracture healing monitoring (Chapter 9), and for that reason it is subject of attention in this book.

Figure 7.5 illustrates the propagation of a spherical wave in the fluid (medium 1 - fluid) towards the solid (medium 2 - solid), with $c_1 < c_2$ (c_1 and c_2 are the ultrasound velocities in media 1 and 2, respectively), generating the lateral wave. It can be determined a critical angle θ_c using the relation

$$\sin(\theta_c) = \frac{c_1}{c_2}. \tag{7.78}$$

When the wavefront reaches the interface, it gives rise to a reflected and refracted wavefront (Figure 7.5(b)). While the incidence angle θ_I is less than θ_c, the point I which connects the direct and reflected wavefronts also connects them with the refracted wavefront. As time passes, the point I moves along the interface with a velocity $v(I)$ defined by

$$v(I) = \frac{c_1}{\sin(\theta_I)}, \tag{7.79}$$

with $v(I) > c_2$. When $\theta_I > \theta_c$, $v(I)$ becomes less than c_2. Hence, the point I does not connect the refracted and reflected wavefronts anymore. The wave that links the refracted to the reflected wavefronts is named lateral wave, as shown in Figure 7.5(c), and it propagates with velocity

$$v_{LW} = \frac{c_1}{\sin(\theta_c)} = c_2. \tag{7.80}$$

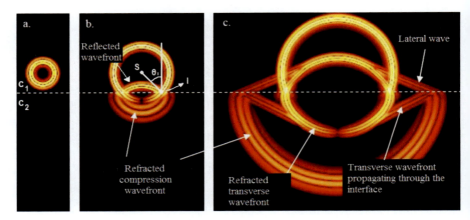

Figure 7.5. (a) Simulation of a spherical wave propagating in a fluid (medium 1) towards a solid (medium 2); (b) when the direct wave reaches the interface fluid-solid, it produces a reflected and a refracted wavefront which are connected by point I, forming a center S and an incidence angle θ_I; (c) when $\theta_I > \theta_c$, the lateral wave is generated (Courtesy from Dr. Emmanuel Bossy - Institut Langevin, ESPCI ParisTech, Paris, France).

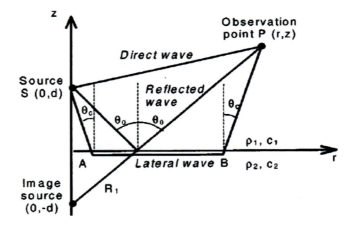

Figure 7.6. Representation of the direct, reflected and lateral waves: SA is the distance between the source S and the point A; BP is the distance between the point B and the observation point P; AB is the distance between the points A and B, ρ_1 and ρ_2 are the densities from media 1 and 2, respectively; r is the distance between the transmitter and the receiver along the interface; d and z are the distances between the source and the observation point until the interface (Reprinted with permission from The Journal of the Acoustical Society of America, vol. 108, n. 6, Estelle Camus, Maryline Talmant, Geneviève Berger, Pascal Laugier, Analysis of the axial transmission technique for the assessment of skeletal status, p. 3059, Copyright (2000), Acoustic Society of America).

Considering Figure 7.6, the pressure of the lateral wave P_{LW} is given by (Camus et al., 2000)

$$P_{LW} = 2i\frac{c_1}{c_2}\left[k_1\frac{\rho_2}{\rho_1}\left(1-\frac{c_1^2}{c_2^2}\right)\sqrt{r}\left[r-(z+d)\tan\theta_c\right]^{3/2}\right]^{-1} \times e^{ik_1\left(SA+BP+\left[c_1/c_2\right]AB\right)}, \quad (7.81)$$

where SA is the distance between the source S and the point A; BP is the distance between the point B and the observation point P; AB is the distance between the points A and B, ρ_1 and ρ_2 are the densities from media 1 and 2, respectively; r is the distance between the transmitter and the receiver along the interface; d and z are the distances between the source and the observation point until the interface. The lateral wave is excited at a critical angle (SA), propagates along the interface (AB) with a longidutinal velocity c_2 and comes back to medium 1 at a critical angle BP.

The lateral wave is only observable beyond a critical point which is localized at a critical range r_c, given by (Camus et al., 2000)

$$r_c = (z+d)\tan(\theta_c). \quad (7.82)$$

Then, the equations of the direct, reflected and lateral times-of-arrival are, respectively

$$t_{DW} = \frac{\left[r^2+(z-d)^2\right]^{1/2}}{c_1}, \quad (7.83)$$

$$t_{RW} = \frac{\left[r^2+(z+d)^2\right]^{1/2}}{c_1} \quad (7.84)$$

and

$$t_{LW} = \frac{r}{c_2} + \frac{(z+d)}{c_1}\left(1-\frac{c_1^2}{c_2^2}\right)^{1/2}. \quad (7.85)$$

It can be shown that the lateral wave will always reach the receptor before the direct wave for values of r greater than r_{min}, defined as

$$r_{min} = (1-\psi^2)^{-1/2} \left[\psi(z+d) + 2(zd)^{1/2} \right] \tag{7.86}$$

where $\psi = c_1/c_2$. Figure 7.7 shows the curves for t_{DW}, t_{RW} and t_{LW}, considering $c_1 = 1490$ m/s and $c_2 = 2680$ m/s.

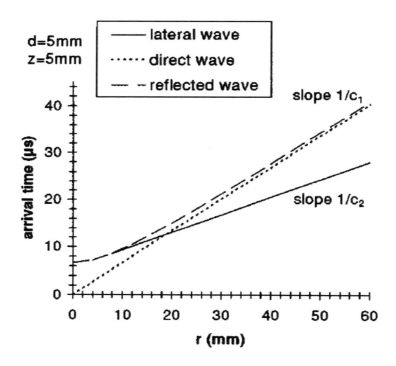

Figure 7.7. Theoretical times-of-arrival for the direct, reflected and lateral waves, considering $c_1 = 1490$ m/s and $c_2 = 2680$ m/s. (Reprinted with permission from The Journal of the Acoustical Society of America, vol. 108, n. 6, Estelle Camus, Maryline Talmant, Geneviève Berger, Pascal Laugier, Analysis of the axial transmission technique for the assessment of skeletal status, p. 3060, Copyright (2000), Acoustic Society of America).

An extension of this problem was studied by Bossy et al. (2002), who considered an infinite solid plate immersed in water (water - solid - water). Figure 7.8 represents this situation.

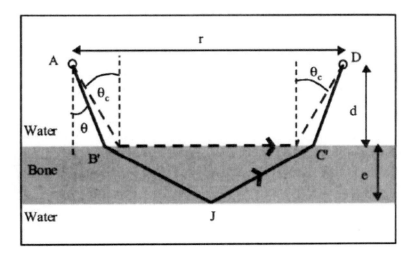

Figure 7.8. Wave trajectories for the lateral wave (dotted line) and the reflected wave from the bottom of the plate (solid line) (Reprinted with permission from The Journal of the Acoustical Society of America, vol. 112, n. 1, Emmanuel Bossy, Maryline Talmant, Pascal Laugier, Effect of bone cortical thickness on velocity measurements using ultrasonic axial transmission: A 2D simulation study, p. 299, Copyright (2002), Acoustic Society of America).

Now, we need to consider the path $AB'JC'D$, which involves only longitudinal waves, and corresponds to a single reflexion from the bottom of the plate (the fast trajectory inside the plate). For a given receptor at a distance r from the source, the incidence angle θ of a wave propagating through the path $AB'JC'D$ and with an associated time-of-flight $t_{AB'JC'D}$, it is possible to yield the following equations (Bossy et al., 2002):

$$t_{AB'JC'D} = \frac{2d}{c_1} \times \frac{1}{\cos(\theta_c)} + \frac{2e}{c_2} \times \frac{1}{\sqrt{1-\left(\frac{sen(\theta)}{sen(\theta_c)}\right)^2}} \tag{7.87}$$

and

$$r = 2d\tan(\theta) + 2e \frac{sen(\theta)}{sen(\theta_c)} \times \frac{1}{\sqrt{1-\left(\frac{sen(\theta)}{sen(\theta_c)}\right)^2}} \tag{7.88}$$

where e is the plate thickness. The difference $t_{AB'JC'D} - t_{LW}$ depends on the distance r and the thickness e. For plates thick enough (typically $e > \lambda$), the velocity of the lateral wave is independent from e, for several distances r and wave detection criteria. For thinner plates (typically $e \leq \lambda$), variations in lateral wave velociry depend on detection criteria and distance r. Nevertheless, for plates too much thin (typically $e \leq \lambda/8$), and for amplitude-independent detection criteria, the lateral wave velocity is similar to that of S0 Lamb mode velocity. According to Bossy et al. (2002), for cortical bone with thickness less than $\lambda/4$, an approach with Lamb waves is necessary.

Conclusion

Ultrasound propagation in bones is very complex. It involves different wave types and interaction mechanisms (absorption, scattering, mode conversion) between the wave and the tissue, and it critically depends on skeletal parameters and experimental conditions.

It can also be concluded that the analysis of wave propagation in cortical bone is much easier than in trabecular bone, because the former can be considered as a homogeneous medium in lower frequency ranges, acting as a simple waveguide. On the other hand, further research is needed to completely elucidate how acoustic waves travel through bone tissue, and how quantitative parameters can be better interpreted.

This chapter ends the first section of this book, which aimed at presenting some basic theoretical background about bone tissue (biology, biomechanics, fracture healing), acoustic wave propagation, acoustic transducers, ultrasound scattering and imaging, and ultrasound propagation in bone. The next section converges all this knowledge to discuss scientific evidences about how ultrasound can be used for both assessment (Chapters 8 and 9) and therapy (Chapters 10 and 11) in bone fractures.

References

Auld, B. A. (1973). *Acoustic Fields and Waves in Solids: Volume I* (1st edition). New York: John Wiley & Sons.

Biot, M. A. (1956). The theory of propagation of elastic waves in fluid-saturated porous solid. I. Low frequency range. *Journal of the Acoustical Society of America, 28*, 168-178.

Biot, M. A. (1956). The theory of propagation of elastic waves in fluid-saturated porous solid. I. Higher frequency range. *Journal of the Acoustical Society of America, 28*, 179-191.

Bossy, E., Talmant, M., & Laugier, P. (2002). Effect of bone cortical thickness on velocity measurements using ultrasonic axial transmission: A 2D simulation study. *Journal of the Acoustical Society of America, 112*, 297-307.

Camus, E., Talmant, M., Berger, G., & Laugier, P. (2000). Analysis of the axial transmission technique for the assessment of skeletal status. *Journal of the Acoustical Society of America, 108*, 3058-3065.

Cobbold, R. S. C. (2007). *Foundations of Biomedical Ultrasound* (1st edition). Oxford: Oxford University Press.

Faran, J. J. (1951). Sound scattering by solid cylinders and spheres. *Journal of the Acoustical Society of America, 23*, 405-418.

Fellah, Z. E. A., Depollier, C., & Fellah, M. (2001). An approach to direct and inverse time-domain scattering of acoustic waves from rigid porous materials by a fractional calculus based method. *Journal of Sound and Vibration, 244*, 359-366.

Fellah, Z. E. A., Sebaa, N., Fellah, M., Mitri, F. G., Ogam, E., Lauriks, W., & Depollier, C. (2008). Application of the Biot model to ultrasound in bone: direct problem. *IEEE Transactions on Ultrasonics, Ferroeletrics, and Frequency Control, 55*, 1508-1515.

Haire, T. J., & Langton, C. M. (1999). Biot theory: A review of its application on ultrasound propagation through cancellous bone. *Bone, 24*, 291–295.

Hosokawa, A., & Otani, T. (1997). Ultrasonic wave propagation in bovine cancellous bone. *Journal of the Acoustical Society of America, 101*, 558–562.

Hosokawa, A., & Otani, T. (1998). Acoustic anisotropy in bovine cancellous bone. *Journal of the Acoustical Society of America*, 103, 2718–2722.

Hughes, E. R., Leighton, T. G., Petley, G. W., White, P. R., & Chivers, R. C. (2003). Estimation of critical and viscous frequencies for Biot theory in cancellous bone. *Ultrasonics, 41*, 365-368.

Johnson, D. L., Koplik, J., & Dashen, R. (1987). Theory of dynamic permeability and tortuosity in fluid-saturated porous media. *Journal of Fluid Mechanics, 176*, 379-402.

Kaczmarek, M., Kubik, J., & Pakula, M. (2002). Short ultrasonic waves in cancellous bone. *Ultrasonics, 46*, 95-100.

Lee, K. I., & Yoon, S. W. (2006). Comparison of acoustic characteristics predicted by Biot's theory and the modified Biot-Attenborough model in cancellous bone. *Journal of Biomechanics, 39*, 364-368.

Moilanen, P., Talmant, M., Kilappa, V., Nicholson, P., Cheng, S., Timonen, J., & Laugier, P. (2008). Modeling the impact of soft tissue on axial transmission measurements of ultrasonic guided waves in human radius. *Journal of the Acoustical Society of America, 124*, 2364-2373.

Morse, P. M., & Ingard, K. U. (1987). *Theoretical Acoustics*. Princeton: Princeton University Press.

Padilla, F., & Wear, K. (2011). Scattering by Trabecular Bone. In: P. Laugier, & G. Haïat (Eds.), *Bone Quantitative Ultrasound* (1st edition, pp. 83-121). New York, NY: Springer.

Padilla, F., Peyrin, F., & Laugier, P. (2003). Prediction of backscatter coefficient in trabecular bones using a numerical model of three-dimensional microstructure. *Journal of the Acoustical Society of America, 113*, 1122-1129.

Pakula, M., Padilla, F., Laugier, P. (2009). Influence of the filling fluid on frequency-dependent velocity and attenuation in cancellous bone between 0.35 and 2.5 MHz. *Journal of the Acoustical Society of America, 126*, 3301-3310.

Pakula, M., Kaczmarek, M., & Padilla, F. (2011). Poromechanical Models. In: P. Laugier, & G. Haïat (Eds.), *Bone Quantitative Ultrasound* (1st edition, pp. 83-121). New York, NY: Springer.

Protopappas, V. C., Fotiadis, D. I., & Malizos, K. N. (2006). Guided ultrasound wave propagation in intact and healing long bones. *Ultrasound in Medicine & Biology, 32*, 693-708.

Protopappas, V. C., Kourtis, I. C., Kourtis, L. C., Malizos, K. N., Massalas, C. V., & Fotiadis, D. I. (2007). Three-dimensional finite element modeling of guided ultrasound wave propagation in intact and healing long bones. *Journal of the Acoustical Society of America, 121*, 3907–3921.

Sebaa, N., Fellah, Z. E. A., Fellah, M., Ogam, E., Mitri, F. G., Depollier, C., & Lauriks, W. Application of the Biot model to ultrasound in bone: inverse problem. *IEEE Transactions on Ultrasonics, Ferroeletrics, and Frequency Control, 55*, 1516-1523.

Talmant, M., Kolta, S., Roux, C., Haguenauer, D., Vedel, I., Cassou, B., Bossy, E., & Laugier, P. (2009). *In vivo* performance evaluation of bi-directional ultrasonic axial transmission for cortical bone assessment. *Ultrasound in Medicine & Biology, 35*, 912-919.

Wilson, J. L. (1992). Ultrasonic wave propagation in cancellous bone and cortical bone: prediction of some experimental results by Biot's theory. *Journal of the Acoustical Society of America, 91*, 1106–1112.

Section III – Ultrasound as a Clinical Assessment Tool for Fracture Healing

Chapter 8

Ultrasound Imaging and Bone Fractures

Abstract

Ultrasound B-mode imaging (ultrasonography) is not the gold standard diagnostic tool in daily clinical practice for fracture assessment. However, it can show poorly ossified tissues better than radiographs, and it is a nonionizing, low-cost and easily operated diagnostic device. Portability can also be another great advantage of ultrasonography. Because there is a decrease in amplitude and intensity as the acoustic waves travel through the tissue, ultrasonography may be suitable only for superficial fractures. The number of publications has increased in the last years, and some clinical situations in which ultrasound shows to be useful are facial traumas, rib and sternum fractures, neonatal care and in emergency departments (ED's). Diagnostic criteria for fracture diagnosis have been discontinuity or irregularity of the cortical line, cortical depression, periosteal elevations, and the presence of subperiosteal fluid collection. When compared to conventional radiographs or computed tomography, ultrasonography presents satisfactory degrees of accuracy, sensitivity and specificity.

8.1. Introduction

Bone fractures can take place in various anatomical sites, from skull, spine and thoracic wall, to upper and lower limbs. It was stated in a previous chapter that acoustic waves are highly attenuated by bone; this may be one of the reasons why ultrasound would not be a suitable diagnostic tool for fractures. With the help of a good anatomy textbook or atlas, we may identify several layers of soft tissues (muscle, fat, vessels, tendons, fasciae, skin) around bones, for example, in arms, legs and some regions of the hip bone. These tissues interact with ultrasound mainly by: (1) absorbing ultrasound energy along its path; and (2) scattering the acoustic energy in the interfaces of tissues. Consequently, the acoustic energy is attenuated until it reaches cortical bone, and its scattering is not sufficient to generate an adequate image for diagnostic purposes. Nevertheless, ultrasound imaging can at least be more applicable to superficial fracture sites.

In chapter 3, the fracture healing phenomenon was introduced. Before anything else, a fracture hematoma is formed, and then the secondary fracture healing combines intramembranous and endochondral ossification to generate the callus, which will be progressively mineralized for some weeks. Clinically available ultrasound imaging techniques are still not capable to adequately assess the callus formation (phases of healing) and remodeling. *In vitro* and *in vivo* methods in animal models are already published by the scientific community, but further investigation is needed.

The aim of this chapter is to present the utilization of ultrasound B-mode imaging for bone fracture assessment. It is intended to show some examples for intact bones before discussing the evidences for fracture healing monitoring.

8.2. Bone Ultrasound B-Mode Imaging

Chapter 6 explored the ultrasound B-mode imaging, a series of A-mode lines received by transducer elements inside a probe, put one beside the other to form an image. Echo amplitudes are used to set gray-scale values, for example, white for maximum echo amplitude, and black for echo amplitude zero. Here some B-mode images in which intact cortical bone can be identified are shown.

Figure 8.1 shows B-mode imaging of the long head tendon of the biceps brachii muscle (a two-headed muscle of the arm, with each muscle bundle with its own origin near the elbow joint). The long head tendon originates from the supraglenoid tubercle (above the shoulder joint) and it passes down along the intertubercular groove of the humerus (Gilroy et al., 2012; Moore et al., 2012). Five important aspects which are worth highlighting: (1) the small white arrows (mouse pointers from the ultrasound equipment) indicates the long head tendon; (2) just under the tendon, the humerus (cortical bone) can be identified; (3) a layer of soft tissue (fat, skin) above the tendon can be observed; (4) the acoustic shadowing under the humerus can be seen (bone works as a strong absorbing material, blocking the passage of sound waves); and (5) "speckle" is present in the image (a granular texture filling the biological structures). As the sound waves reach the interfaces between tissues, they are reflected with a magnitude proportional to the acoustic impedance mismatch (Chapter 4). Cortical bone is usually well defined in ultrasound images (high impedance compared to soft tissues), but nothing else can be evaluated more internally (acoustic shadowing).

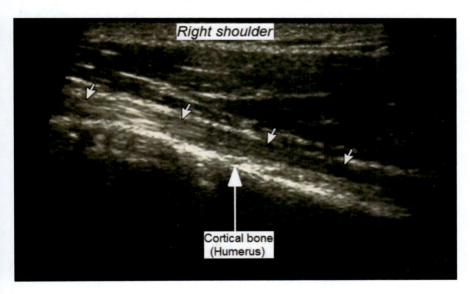

Figure 8.1. B-mode imaging of the long head tendon of the right biceps brachii muscle (small white arrows). The cortical layer of humerus and the acoustic shadowing can be identified (Courtesy from Prof. Carlos Alberto V. de Melo - Physical Therapy Department - Estácio de Sá University - Nova Friburgo, Rio de Janeiro, Brazil).

Figure 8.2 shows an image of the subscapularis tendon of a patient with calcific tendonitis (formation of small calcium deposits within the tendon). The subscapularis muscle arises from the subscapular fossa of the scapula and inserts into the lesser tubercle of the humerus and the anterior part of the shoulder joint capsule (Gilroy et al., 2012; Moore et al., 2012). It forms part of posterior wall of axila (Bradley and O'Donnell, 2002). The small white arrows indicate the calcium deposits. Other detectable structures are: (1) the subscapularis tendon; (2) the deltoid muscle around the humerus; (3) a cross-section view of the long head tendon of the biceps brachii muscle; and (4) the cortical layer of humerus in two important muscular insertion sites: the lesser and greater tuberosities. The acoustic shadowing can be identified below the humerus line.

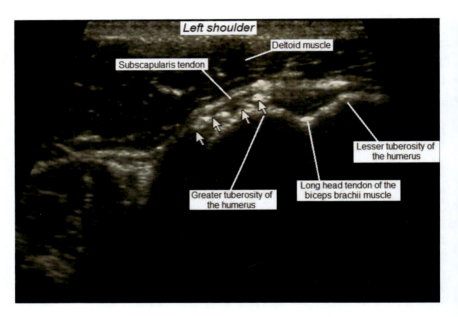

Figure 8.2. B-mode imaging of the subscapularis tendon of a patient with calcific tendonitis. The small calcific deposits within the tendon are shown by the small white arrows. One can also identify the cortical layer of humerus (lesser and greater tuberosities), the deltoid muscle, a cross-section view of the long head tendon of the biceps brachii muscle, and the acoustic shadowing below the humerus line (Courtesy from Prof. Carlos Alberto V. de Melo - Physical Therapy Department - Estácio de Sá University - Nova Friburgo, Rio de Janeiro, Brazil).

A B-mode image from the calcaneal tendon can be seen in Figure 8.3. It is a tendon of the posterior leg, attaching the gastrocnemius, soleus and plantaris muscles to the calcaneus bone. Again the acoustic shadowing produced by the bone can also be observed. The tendon is easily identified.

Interesting pictures are shown in Figure 8.4. They are B-mode images from a child who had a knee injury. It is possible to see a large collection of fluid or hematoma (H) in the suprapatellar region, due to a formation of hemorrhagic effusion which may extend into the suprapatellar bursa. The hematoma can be observed above the patella, deep to the quadriceps tendon and superficial to the distal portion of femur. Note the acoustic shadowing under the cortical boundary of patella and femur.

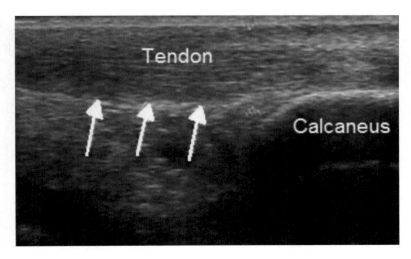

Figure 8.3. B-mode imaging of the calcaneal tendon (arrows). The cortical region of calcaneus bone and the acoustic shadowing under it can be identified (Courtesy from Prof. Carlos Alberto V. de Melo - Physical Therapy Department - Estácio de Sá University - Nova Friburgo, Rio de Janeiro, Brazil).

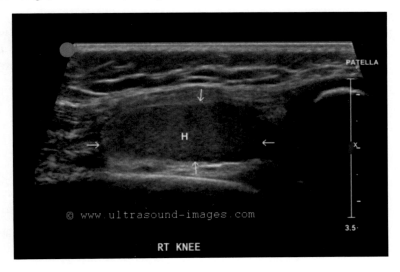

Figure 8.4. B-mode image from a child after a traumatic knee injury. A collection of fluid or hematoma (H) in the suprapatellar region can be identified (Reprinted from http://www.ultrasound-images.com, with permission from Dr. Joe Antony, MD).

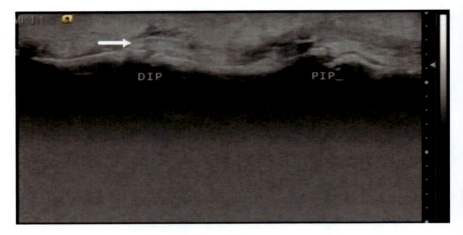

Figure 8.5. B-mode image of the 4th finger of a young boy who suffered a sports injury. The white arrow indicates a rupture of the tendon of the flexor digitorum profundus muscle. DIP = distal interphalngeal joint; PIP = proximal interphalangeal joint (Figure 8.4. B-mode image from a child after a traumatic knee injury. A collection of fluid or hematoma (H) in the suprapatellar region can be identified (Reprinted from http://www.ultrasound-images.com, with permission from Dr. Joe Antony, MD).

The right 4th finger of a young boy who suffered a sports injury is shown in Figure 8.5. One can observe a rupture or avulsion of the tendon of the flexor digitorum profundus muscle (white arrow). This condition is called a Jersey finger and it is the result of acute injury to the distal phalanx resulting in sudden forced extension of the affected finger when it is flexed. The distal interphalngeal joint (DIP) and proximal interphalangeal joint (PIP) are also indicated.

8.3. Ultrasound B-Mode Imaging and Bone Fractures

The ultrasound B-mode imaging (ultrasonography) is not the gold standard diagnostic tool in daily clinical practice for fracture assessment. On the other hand, radiography is still an exam of choice since it is relatively inexpensive and provides an infinity of assessment possibilities: bone and joint alignment, joint spacing, bone texture, bone fractures, cortical outline, and to some extent soft tissues. Bone contains calcium (an atom with a high atomic number), thus efficiently absorbing X-rays. The amount of X-rays arriving at the detector will be reduced in the shadow of bones, making it clearly visible on the radiograph. Fracture lines are often easily identifiable in this imaging mode.

Although ultrasound may show poorly ossified tissues better than radiographs, and it lacks ionizing radiation. There is a decrease in amplitude and intensity as the acoustic waves travel through the tissue. For this reason, ultrasonography is not adequate for fractures in bones surrounded by a dense volume of muscles or other soft tissues. Nevertheless, there are some medical applications of ultrasound imaging showing to be useful, for example, in facial traumas, rib and sternum fractures, neonatal care and emergency departments (ED's), and the number of publications has increased in the last years.

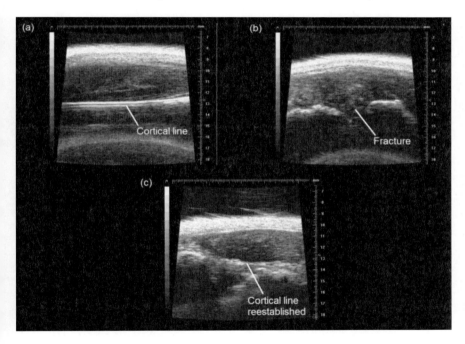

Figure 8.6. High-resolution ultrasonography of an adult Wistar rat femur: (a) intact femur; (b) after a surgical intervention, leading to a pseudoarthrosis; and (c) cortical line reestablished after a treatment protocol (Courtesy from Prof. Dr. Célia Resende - Federal University of Rio de Janeiro - Brazil).

First of all, let us take a look on an ultrasonography of an intact and a fractured femur from an adult Wistar rat, using a high-resolution equipment (30 MHz). In Figure 8.6(a), it is possible to identify the cortical line of the intact femur. After a surgical procedure followed by a model for pseudoarthrosis development (a failed bone regeneration, leading to an unhealed area with motion), the space between the bone fragments can be observed in Figure 8.6(b) since the ultrasound beam is not reflected and it penetrates into the fracture gap. Finally, after a treatment protocol, the cortical line was reestablished, as seen in Figure 8.6(c), despite the abnormal alignment. This example of an animal model shows that ultrasonography may be able to detect cortical discontinuities, as well as bone regeneration on a more superficial site. However, it is very difficult to evaluate deeper regions or even the mechanical properties of callus (stiffness, for example).

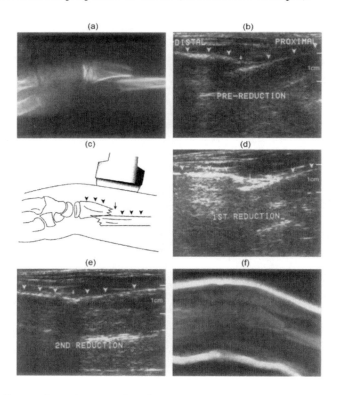

Figure 8.7. Images from the case of an 8-year-old girl with a right forearm fracture. The large arrows indicate the dorsal cortex of radius, and the small arrow indicates the fracture site: (a) lateral radiograph of forearm; (b) B-mode ultrasound image in plane anterior-posterior showing the displaced fracture; (c) a schematic diagram showing the position of ultrasound transducer during assessment; (d) B-mode ultrasound image showing persistent displacement after a first attempt to reduction; (e) B-mode ultrasound image after a second reduction indicating a good alignment; (f) a radiograph after the second reduction and splinting (Reprinted from The American Journal of Emergency Medicine, vol. 18, n. 1, William Durston, Richard Swarzentruber, Ultrasound guided reduction of pediatric forearm fractures in the ED, p. 73, Copyright (2000) with permission from W.B./Saunders Co.).

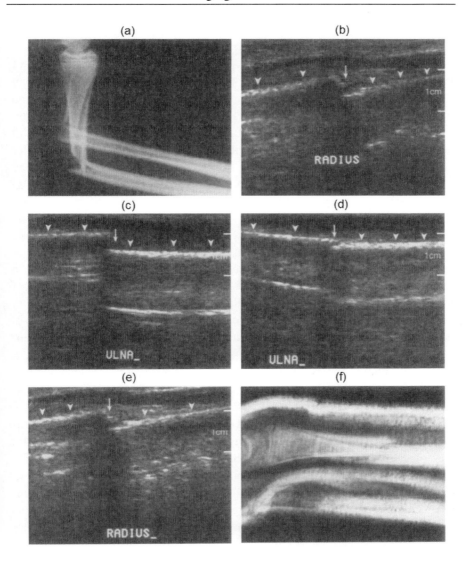

Figure 8.8. Images from the case of a 16-year-old boy with a left forearm deformity. The large arrows indicate the dorsal cortex, and the small arrow indicates the fracture site: (a) a lateral radiograph shows the displaced fractures of distal radius and ulna; (b) B-mode ultrasound image of distal radius after the first reduction; (c) B-mode ultrasound image of ulna after the first reduction; (d) B-mode ultrasound image after the second reduction; (e) B-mode ultrasound image of radius after the second reduction; (f) a lateral radiograph after splinting (Reprinted from The American Journal of Emergency Medicine, vol. 18, n. 1, William Durston, Richard Swarzentruber, Ultrasound guided reduction of pediatric forearm fractures in the ED, p. 76, Copyright (2000) with permission from W.B./Saunders Co.).

It is possible to find some scientific evidence from literature concerning the application of ultrasonography in fracture diagnosis. In 2000, Durston and Swartzentruber presented three case histories showing the usefulness of bedside ultrasound (BUS) to guide reduction of pediatric forearm fractures in an emergency department (ED). Figure 8.7 shows radiographs, ultrasound images and a schematic diagram from a case of an 8-year-old girl with a right forearm fracture. The radiograph and B-mode image, as seen in Figures 8.7(a) and 8.7(b), respectively, indicate a displaced fracture of the distal radius. After anesthesia, a first attempt to reduce the fracture was done, and the result can be seen in Figure 8.7(d) as a persistent misalignment. A second attempt to reduction was performed, and the correct alignment was obtained (Figure 8.7(e)). A radiograph confirmed the satisfactory result (Figure 8.7(f)). The same study described another case of a 16-year-old young man with a visible left arm deformity after falling from a tree. A markedly displaced fracture of the distal radius and ulna can be seen in the radiograph (Figure 8.8(a)). After a first attempt to reduction, the angulation was corrected but there was still a persistent dorsal displacement of both the distal radius (Figure 8.8(b)) and ulna (Figure 8.8(c)). A second attempt to reduction was done, the ulna was completely corrected (Figure 8.8(d)) however with a persistent misalignment in the distal radius (Figure 8.8(e)), which was also demonstrated with a radiograph (Figure 8.8(f)). Years later, Chaar-Alvarez et al. (2011) obtained an overall accuracy of 94% in the diagnosis of pediatric distal forearm fractures, with a sensitivity and specificity of 96% and 93%, respectively.

Bruno et al. (2008) aimed at assessing the accuracy of radiography and ultrasonography in defining both the distance between the bone edges and the rate and quality of callus formation in distraction osteogenesis of the mandible in a series of patients. In this surgical technique, a corticotomy is used to fracture the bone into two segments which are gradually moved apart during the distraction phase, leading to bone formation in the gap. It is used to reconstruct skeletal deformities and lengthen the long bones of the body. The results demonstrated that the ultrasound beam (as discussed before in this chapter) is not reflected before the development of a new cortical line, and it can penetrate into the fracture gap. As fracture healing takes place, small echogenic islands may appear, progressively increasing in volume, leading to a decrease in ultrasound beam penetration depth. After 30-80 days of fixation, bone continuity is finally restored, and one can observe the onset of a beam-reflecting hyperechoic surface and the formation of an acoustic shadowing. The interobserver agreement was high, although the assessment of callus maturity was subjectively made.

Park et al. (2009) proposed the use of 10-MHz ultrasonography as an intraoperative repositioning control of nasal bone fractures in 32 patients. Radiographs and computed tomography were also used. All the cases were clearly detected by ultrasound imaging. A value of 100% for sensitivity and positive predictive value was obtained, confirming the usefulness of this technique for the assessment of facial bone fractures.

Simanovsky et al. (2009) developed a prospective experiment to determine the effectiveness of ultrasound (5-12 MHz) in differentiating radiographically occult fractures from ankle or wrist sprains. Follow-up radiographs were made between 2 and 3 weeks after injury, and compared with the initial radiographs. Fifty-eight patients participated in this study, ranging between the ages of 2 to 16. Ultrasound was able to identify small metaphyseal cortical fractures of the distal fibula in 17 patients, since one or more of the following signs were present in the image: (1) a discontinuity of the cortical line, (2) cortical depression, (3) small echogenic fragment adjacent to the cortex, (4) a periosteal elevation, and (5) the presence of subperiosteal fluid collection.

Ang et al. (2010) studied the effectiveness of ultrasound guidance in the reduction of distal radius fractures in adult patients. They compared a prospective cohort of patients in which ultrasound was used to guide fracture reductions, with a retrospective group of patients in which these proceduress were done with blind manual palpation. Figure 8.7 shows the B-mode images before and after fracture manipulation and reduction. The repeated attempts at manipulations and reductions were significantly reduced using ultrasound. From the 62 patients belonging to the ultrasound group, only one (1.6%) required another attempt. In the control group, 9 patients were submitted to more than one reduction attempt (8.8%), although this difference was not significant ($p = 0.056$). However, when comparing rates of surgical intervention, 4.9% of the patients in the ultrasound group required open reduction and internal fixation for the management of their fractures, whereas 16.7% in the control group required this procedure ($p = 0.02$).

Weinberg et al. (2010) evaluated the test performance characteristics of clinically-performed point-of-care ultrasound (7.5-10 MHz), comparing the results to radiography or CT scans, for the diagnosis of pediatric long and non-long bone fractures. A total of 212 patients underwent ultrasound assessments (with 348 bones imaged) with a median age of 13 years old. The presence/absence of cortical interruption or irregularity was used as an assessment criterion, as shown in Figure 8.10. With one hour of ultrasound training sessions with novice sonographers, it was possible to assure a high degree of accuracy in the diagnosis of long and non-long bone fractures (there was no statistical significant difference in accuracy between long and non-long bones assessment). The main cause of errors in this study (a total of 12.35%) was the location of fractures near the epiphysis of long bones or near joints, because of irregular contours. Other errors were obtained, for example: in a fractured clavicular shaft, a fractured phalanx shaft, a fractured mandibular ramus, false positive sonograms (X-ray negative) of a rib and phalanx, and a midshaft fracture of ulna.

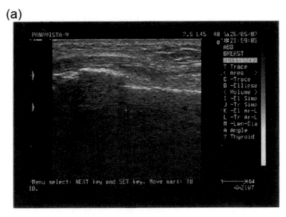

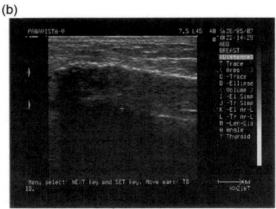

Figure 8.9. Ultrasonography of distal radius from an adult patient. (a) and (b) show, respectively, the image before and after manipulation and reduction (Reprinted from The American Journal of Emergency Medicine, vol. 28, n. 9, Shiang-Hu Ang, Shu-Woan Lee, Kai-Yet Lam, Ultrasound-guided reduction of distal radius fractures, p. 1004, Copyright (2010) with permission from Elsevier).

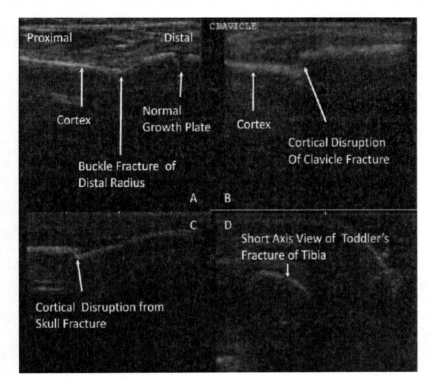

Figure 8.10. B-mode images of fractures from the study of Weinberg et al. (2010): (a) a buckle fracture of distal radius (incomplete fracture of the shaft of a long bone, with bulging of the cortex); (b) a clavicle fracture; (c) a skull fracture; (d) a Toddler's fracture of tibia (undisplaced spiral fractures) (Reprinted from Injury, vol. 41, n. 8, Eric Weinberg, Michael Tunik, James Tsung, Accuracy of clinician-performed point-of-care ultrasound for the diagnosis of fractures in children and young adults, p. 864, Copyright (2010) with permission from Elsevier).

A comparison BUS x radiography was also made by Cross et al. (2010) for clavicle fractures in patients aging from 1 to 18 years old. A 10-15 MHz ultrasound device was used to visualize the clavicle bone starting at the sternal junction and moving laterally. Then radiographs were taken as ordered by the attending emergency physician. It was found to be a good to excellent interrater reliability (kappa = 0.74, 95% CI = 0.60 to 0.88). The authors made an interesting observation: clavicle fractures are excellent applications for novice ultrasonographers in emergency rooms, since the patients are usually stable; the procedure is rapid, easy to perform and to interpret. Some limitations of the study were the small number of researchers at a single department, a convenience sample, and the absence of a follow-up after patient discharge (occult clavicle fractures diagnosed after the initial presentation may have been missed). Chien et al. (2011) also focused on clavicle fractures from a convenience sample of 58 patients younger than 17 years old, obtaining a sensitivity of 89.7% and a specificity of 89.5%.

The detection of rib fractures were the goal of Turk et al. (2010). A total of 20 patients with blunt chest trauma participated in this study. A 12-MHz ultrasound device was used. Analysis with radiographs did not detect any fracture. On the contrary, ultrasonography identified 26 rib fractures in 90% of the patients. The authors discussed important issues in this clinical situation: (1) it may be a very hard task to image subscapular ribs and the infraclavicular portion of the first rib; (2) the sonographer may be confused by the pleura, which has a similar sonographic appearance to the rib cortex; and (3) if the transducer is not entirely laid over the rib, pseudofractures can be produced in the image.

You et al. (2010) evaluated the performance of ultrasonography in sternal fractures. Thirty-six patients were enrolled in the study, with recent chest trauma. After a radiographic analysis, the B-mode images were obtained using a transducer with frequency 7-12 MHz. The radiologist was blinded to the results of the other test. An abrupt discontinuity of the bone surface with or without a step-off deformity was used as a diagnostic criterion. A sensitivity of 70.8% and specificity of 75.0% for conventional radiographs was found ; however, the sensitivity and specificity of ultrasonography were both 100%.

The U.S. Military Forces have already proposed ultrasound as an important ally in decision making inside battlefields. Vasios et al. (2010) presented four case reports as an example of ultrasound imaging application in a military combat theater: (1) femur fracture; (2) distal fibular fracture; (3) phalanx fracture; and (4) tibial fracture. Portability, easy availability, simple operation and low-cost devices were the positive aspects demonstrated by the authors. Another study simulated a model for the ultrasound diagnosis of long bone fractures to verify the ability of U.S. Army Special Forces Medics to detect fractures with portable equipment (Heiner et al., 2010). A simple simulation model was composed of a bare turkey leg bone housed in a container within a gelatin solution, with five created patterns: intact bone, transverse, segmental, oblique and comminuted fractures. A sensitivity of 100% and a specificity of 90% was obtained. In spite of the simplicity of this approach, the authors concluded that portable ultrasound would be better explored by military forces. One year later, the same simulation model (Figure 8.11) was used to assess the ability of emergency nurses with minimal training to identify the simulated fractures with an ultrasound device (5-10 MHz) compared to the ability of ED physicians (Heiner et al., 2011).

Emergency nurses were able to diagnose fractures with a high degree of sensitivity and specificity with no significant difference when compared to physicians. Advantages of this approach could be an adjunct to aid in triage dispositions, planning of ED resource utilization and real-time guidance of fracture reduction. B-mode images from this model can be seen in Figure 8.12.

A comparison between the diagnostic utility of BUS and radiography was made by Sinha et al. (2011) to identify long bone fractures in an ED. Forty-one patients were enrolled in the study aging from 7 to 17 years old. Emergency physicians performed sonographic evaluation (7-10 MHz) of the affected region before obtaining a radiograph. Both ultrasonography and radiography were then assessed by a blinded orthopedic specialist. The authors found an overall BUS sensitivity of 89% and a specificity of 100%, and they concluded that BUS can be utilized by emergency physicians after a brief training, with a high degree of accuracy and a rapid diagnostic ability (which is very attractive in busy EDs and when dealing with mass casualties), to identify long bone fractures. A limitation of BUS was the detection of periarticular fractures.

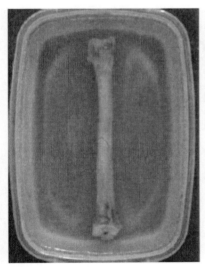
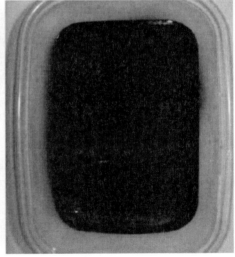

Figure 8.11. Left image: a semi-opaque model used for fracture simulation (turkey leg bone). Right image: an opaque model (Reprinted from International Emergency Nursing, vol. 19, n. 3, Jason Heiner, Aaron Profitt, Todd McArthur, The ability of emergency nurses to detect simulated long bone fractures with portable ultrasound, p. 121, Copyright (2011) with permission from Elsevier).

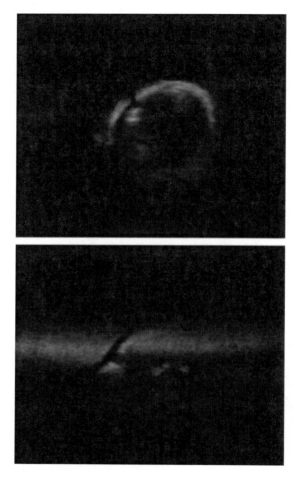

Figure 8.12. B-mode images from the simulated fracture model: transverse axis (top) and long axis (bottom) (Reprinted from International Emergency Nursing, vol. 19, n. 3, Jason Heiner, Aaron Profitt, Todd McArthur, The ability of emergency nurses to detect simulated long bone fractures with portable ultrasound, p. 121, Copyright (2011) with permission from Elsevier).

Adeyemo and Akadiri (2011) reviewed evidences for the use of ultrasonography in maxillofacial fractures. A total of 17 articles, from 1992 to 2009, were selected based on inclusion criteria: two articles considered midfacial fractures, nine considered orbital fractures, three articles considered nasal fractures, two articles considered mandibular fractures, and finally one described case series of ultrasonographic diagnosis of mandibular and midfacial fractures. Despite the high accuracy of ultrasonography in the diagnosis of nasal bone and orbital fractures, several limitations could be detected, for example, the inability to delineate complex multiple facial fractures and to distinguish new fractures from old fractures, confusion in determining the fracture site and difficulty in producing detailed bony imaging due to acute conditions with the presence of extensive oedema. The authors also highlighted factors which may affect the validity of diagnostic ultrasonography in maxillofacial fractures (Table 8.1).

Table 8.1. Factors affecting validity of ultrasonographic diagnosis in maxillofacial fractures (Reprinted from International Journal of Oral and Maxillofacial Surgery, vol. 40, W. L. Adeyemo, O. A. Akadiri, A systematic review of the diagnosis role of ultrasonography in maxillofacial fractures, p. 659, Copyright (2011) with permission from Churchill Livingstone)

1. Experience of sonographer
2. Type and resolution of transducer
3. Lack of standard scanning technique for the facial skeleton
4. Real time visualization is better than interpretation of hard copy
5. Timing of the sonographic investigation from the time of injury

Javadrashid et al. (2011) compared ultrasonography with computed tomography (CT) in the diagnosis of nasal bone fractures. Forty patients with mid-facial fractures were enrolled in this study, and they underwent 7.5-MHz nasal ultrasonography, which was compared to CT imaging. Ultrasonography obtained a sensitivity of 94.9% and specificity of 100% in comparison with CT. The positive predictive value and negative predictive value were 100% and 95.3%, respectively. The authors also used ultrasonography to evaluate healthy nasal bones, obtaining 100% of accuracy, without any false-positive results. In the same year, Mohammadi and Ghasemi-Rad (2011) obtained a sensitivity and specificity of 97% and 100% for nasal bone fractures diagnosis, respectively, compared with 86% and 87% from CT, and 72% and 73% from conventional radiography.

In a case report of an 81-year-old woman, Pearce and Cobby (2011) tried to detect a radiographically occult fracture of the tibial epiphysis, with correlation to CT imaging using 14-MHz equipment. Longitudinal and transverse images showed defects in the anterior tibial cortex. A CT scan was arranged to confirm the presence of an undisplaced fracture from the tibial epiphysis to the tibial plateau. It was possible to detect cortical discontinuity by ultrasonography.

Platon et al. (2011) assessed ultrasonography (US) performed by an emergency radiologist in 62 patients with normal radiographs but with clinical suspicion of scaphoid fracture. The diagnostic performance of ultrasound resulted in : sensitivity of 92%, specificity of 71%, positive predictive value of 46%, and negative predictive value of 97%. Nonetheless some limitations were pointed out by the authors: not all the scaphoid fractures can be assessed by ultrasonography; the presence of arthritic deformity of the wrist created some confusion to determine cortical irregularities; it is very difficult to discriminate the fluid associated with pathological degenerative processes from the fluid related to fracture; and the presence of fractures in other wrist bones may lead to a false-positive results.

Conclusion

Researchers worldwide have drawn attention to the use of ultrasonography in fracture diagnosis and follow-up in the last couple of years. Conventional radiography and computed tomography (CT) scans are still traditional diagnostic tools, but several drawbacks exist: the superimposition of images of the overlying structures in conventional radiographs, impossibility of a real-time image visualization, limited access to facilities, high cost, and high radiation exposure. In addition, CT requires special subject positioning, which may represent a hard task with uncooperative patients.

The interest in ultrasound as an assessment tool for fractures has been growing, since it is possible to image soft tissues and to render real-time images. Moreover, there is no evidence of possible harm with the use of controlled acoustic intensities, the equipment is relatively inexpensive, and portable equipment is accessible. More common clinical applications seem to be superficial injuries (facial traumas, chest wall traumas, forearm fractures). Ultrasound can show poorly ossified neonatal bones better than radiographs, which is an important factor for neonatal care applications. Evidence suggests several benefits in emergency departments (ED's), for example in triage dispositions and real-time guidance of fracture reduction. Even the military forces have recognized the advantages of using ultrasound equipments in combat theater.

Notwithstanding the above, further research is needed to overcome some limitations. First of all, the reliability of this tool in assessing fractures must be better defined. Care must be taken with the development of a standard sonographic technique for each anatomical site, and the design of special transducer probes. Other disadvantages pointed out by some authors were the difficulty in delineating complex multiple fractures and in analyzing fractures in acute conditions due to the presence of extensive edema. Perhaps the implementation of computer-aided diagnosis (CAD) procedures (already proposed for the diagnosis of breast, lung and colon cancer, coronary disease, and in nuclear medicine) may help physicians better explore ultrasound imaging in the search for bone fractures.

References

Adeyemo, W. L., & Akadiri, O. A. (2011). A systematic review of the diagnostic role of ultrasonography in maxillofacial fractures. *International Journal of Oral & Maxillofacial Surgery, 40,* 655-661.

Ang, S.-H., Lee, S.-W., & Lam, K.-Y. (2010). Ultrasound-guided reduction of distal radius fractures. *The American Journal of Emergency Medicine, 28,* 1002-1008.

Bradley, M., & O'Donnell, P. (2002). *Atlas of Musculoskeletal Ultrasound Anatomy* (1st edition). New York: Cambridge University Press.

Bruno, C., Minniti, S., Buttura-da-Prato, E., Albanese, M., Nocini, P. F., & Pozzi-Mucelli, R. (2008). Gray-scale ultrasonography in the evaluation of bone callus in distraction osteogenesis of the mandible: initial findings. *European Radiology, 18,* 1012-1017.

Chaar-Alvarez, F. M., Warkentine, F., Cross, K., Herr, S., & Paul, R. I. (2011). Bedside ultrasound diagnosis of nonangulated distal forearm fractures in the pediatric emergency department. *Pediatric Emergency Care, 27,* 1027-1032.

Chien, M., Bulloch, B., Garcia-Filion, P., Youssfi, M., Shrader, M. W., & Segal, L. S. (2011). Bedside ultrasound in the diagnosis of pediatric clavicle fractures. *Pediatric Emergency Care, 27,* 1038-1041.

Cross, K. P., Warkentine, F. H., Kim, I. K., Gracely, E., & Paul, R. I. (2010). Bedside Ultrasound Diagnosis of Clavicle Fractures in the Pediatric Emergency Department. *Academic Emergency Medicine, 17,* 687-693.

Durston, W., & Swartzentruber, R. (2000). Ultrasound guided reduction of pediatric forearm fractures in the ED. *American Journal of Emergency Medicine, 18,* 72-77.

Gilroy, A. M., MacPherson, B. R., Ross, L. M., Schuenke, M., Schulte, E., & Schumacher, U. (2012). *Atlas of Anatomy* (2nd edition). New York: Thieme.

Heiner, J. D., Baker, B. L., & McArthur, T. J. (2010). The ultrasound detection of simulated long bone fractures by U.S. Army Special Forces Medics. *Journal of Special Operations Medicine, 10*, 7-10.

Heiner, J. D., Profitt, A. M., & McArthur, T. J. (2011). The ability of emergency nurses to detect simulated long bone fractures with portable ultrasound. *International Emergency Nursing, 19*, 120-124.

Javadrashid, R., Khatoonabad, M. J., Shams, N., Esmaeili, F., & Khamnei, H. J. (2011). Comparison of ultrasonography with computed tomography in the diagnosis of nasal bone fractures. *Dentomaxillofacial Radiology, 40*, 486-491.

Mohammadi, A., & Ghasemi-Rad, M. (2011). Nasal bone fracture-ultrasonography or computed tomography? *Medical Ultrasonography, 13*, 292-295.

Moore, K. L., Dailey, A. F., & Agur, A. M. R. (2012). *Clinically Oriented Anatomy* (6th edition). New York: Lippincott Williams & Wilkins.

Park, C.-H., Joung, H.-H., Lee, J.-H., & Hong, S. M. (2009). Usefulness of ultrasonography in the treatment of nasal bone fractures. *The Journal of Trauma: Injury, Infection and Critical Care, 67*, 1323-1326.

Pearce, T., & Cobby, M. (2011). Radiographically occult fracture of the tibial epiphysis: sonographic findings with CT correlation. *Journal of Clinical Ultrasound, 39*, 425-426.

Platon, A., Poletti, P.-A., Aaken, J. V., Fusetti, C., Santa, D. D., Beaulieu, J.-Y., & Becker, C. D. (2011). Occult fractures of the scaphoid: the role of ultrasonography in the emergency department. *Skeletal Radiology, 40*, 869-875.

Simanovsky, N., Lamdan, R., Hiller, N., & Simanovsky, N. (2009). Sonographic detection of radiographically occult fractures in pediatric ankle and wrist injuries. *Journal of Pediatric Orthopedics, 29*, 142-145.

Sinha, T. P., Bhoi, S., Kumar, S., Ramchandani, R., Goswami, A., Kurrey, L., & Galwankar, S. (2011). Diagnostic accuracy of bedside emergency ultrasound screening for fractures in pediatric trauma patients. *Journal of Emergencies, Trauma and Shock, 4*, 443-445.

Turk, F., Kurt, A. B., & Saglam, S. (2010). Evaluation by ultrasound of traumatic rib fractures missed by radiography. *Emergency Radiology, 17*, 473-477.

Vasios, W. N., Hubler, D. A., Lopez, R. A., & Morgan, A. R. (2010). Fracture detection in a combat theater: four cases comparing ultrasound to conventional radiography. *Journal of Special Operations Medicine, 10*, 11-15.

Weinberg, E. R., Tunik, M. G., & Tsung, J. W. (2010). Accuracy of clinician-performed point-of-care ultrasound for the diagnosis of fractures in children and young adults. *Injury, 41*, 862-868.

You, J. S., Chung, Y. E., Kim, D., Park, S., & Chung, S. P. (2010). Role of sonography in the emergency room to diagnose sternal fractures. *Journal of Clinical Ultrasound, 38*, 135-137.

Chapter 9

Quantitative Ultrasound Techniques and Bone Fractures

Abstract

Quantitative ultrasound (QUS) refers to the quantification of parameters from the transmitted or backscattered ultrasound radio-frequency (RF) signals after its propagation through the biological tissue, and it is passing through a rapid expansion nowadays. QUS has been developed by means of two techniques: the transverse (through-transmission and pulse-echo modes) and axial transmission. In through-transmission mode of transverse transmission technique, a transmitter and a receiver element are used at opposite sides of the studied sample. The pulse-echo mode uses only one transducer, acting as an emitter and receiver, and the sample is placed above a perfect reflector. Finally, the axial transmission (AT) technique, which consists in placing a set of linearly arranged transducers along the bones axis. The receivers detect the ultrasound waves that have been propagated along the cortical shell, and some parameters can be estimated. Some QUS parameters that can be used for tissue characterization are the speed of sound (SOS), the broadband ultrasonic attenuation (BUA), the backscattering coefficient and the mean scatterer spacing (MSS) with transverse transmission modes. In axial transmission, the time-of-flight of the first arriving signal (TOF_{FAS}), the sound pressure level (SPL) and a multi-signal approach with multi-element probes can be applied. Literature has shown several developments on the possibility of QUS application for fracture healing monitoring and assessment, by means of experiments and simulations.

The mechanical and geometric properties of the callus tissue may influence the wave propagation through the fracture gap, providing important information about the fracture healing status.

9.1. Introduction

Ultrasound applications in Medicine have been primarily developed for diagnostic imaging. It is worth remembering the role of the Dussik brothers, the first ones to use acoustic waves for medical purposes, trying to localize brain tumors by through-transmission attenuation images, in 1942.

Together with the technologic evolution in biomedical engineering, another ultrasound approach has been gaining space: the **quantitative ultrasound (QUS)** techniques. It refers to the quantification of parameters from the transmitted or backscattered ultrasound radiofrequency (RF) signals after its propagation through the biological tissue. Examples of QUS parameters are the speed of sound (SOS) (Wear et al., 2008), broadband ultrasound attenuation (BUA) coefficient (Bossy et al., 2007), backscattering coefficient (Jenson et al., 2003), and mean scatterer spacing (MSS) (Machado et al., 2006).

QUS is passing through a rapid expansion nowadays. In 2008, a special volume of the IEEE Transactions on Ultrasonics, Ferroelectrics, and Frequency Control presented several authors from different countries who are researching important topics on this matter. According to Laugier (2008, p. 1179):

> QUS provides an umbrella of techniques that do not just give one parameter, such as the absorption coefficient as in the case of X-rays, but potentially a multitude of variables. Because the ultrasound propagation characteristics are principally determined by structural and material properties of the propagation medium, QUS in principle should allow an advanced assessment of bone strength. However, this potential advantage of ultrasound has not been fully exploited so far because the underlying physical theory is still not completely understood [...]. Nevertheless, in the past 15 years, the field has produced a diversity of innovative technological developments targeting *in vivo* bone strength characterization.

It was just for fracture healing monitoring that QUS began its history. Siegel et al. (1958) measured the speed of sound of a wave propagating in the tibia. Since then developments were made for osteoporosis discrimination (Langton et al., 1984), fracture risk in osteoporotic patients (Marin et al., 2006; Talmant et al., 2009), bone strength evaluation (Litmanovitz et al., 2003; Haïat et al., 2008), and finally the subject of this book, fracture healing assessment.

This chapter will present an introduction to QUS (transverse and axial transmission techniques, QUS parameters commonly used etc.) and some scientific evidences (*in vitro* and *in vivo* studies) about the application of QUS techniques in the assessment of fracture healing process.

9.2. What Is the Difference between Transverse and Axial Transmission Measurements?

QUS has been developed by means of two widely used techniques of ultrasound data acquisition: the **transverse** (through-transmission and pulse-echo modes) and **axial transmission**. All of these methods are usually performed in a water bath. The **through-transmission mode** of transverse transmission technique uses a transmitter and a receiver element, at opposite sides of the studied sample. The method has been applied to measure BUA and SOS at several bones (phalanxes, calcaneus, radius, proximal femur) (Laugier, 2011). Generally, the signal transmitted through the sample and received by the second transducer element (or the time-of-flight - TOF) is compared with the signal transmitted through a reference medium (for example, water), as shown in Figure 9.1.

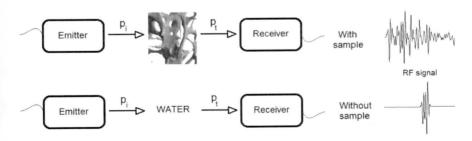

Figure 9.1. The transverse transmission (through-transmission mode) technique: (a) with the bone sample and (b) without the sample. Water is used as the reference medium, and p_i and p_t are, respectively, the incident and the transmitted ultrasound pressure.

The **pulse-echo mode** uses only one transducer, which acts as an emitter and receiver. The sample to be analyzed is placed above a perfect reflector (Figure 9.2). The signal transmitted through the sample reaches the reflector, and turns back to the same transducer. For signal analysis, once again the signal transmitted through the sample is compared with the signal transmitted through the reference (Pereira et al., 2008).

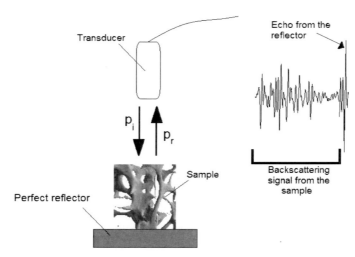

Figure 9.2. The transverse transmission (pulse-echo mode) technique. p_i and p_r are, respectively, the incident and the reflected ultrasound pressure.

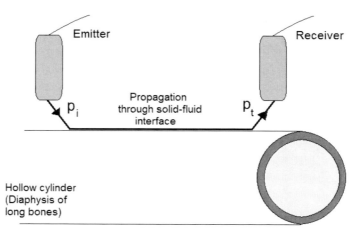

Figure 9.3. The axial transmission technique. p_i and p_t are, respectively, the incident and the transmitted ultrasound pressure.

Finally, the **axial transmission** (AT) technique, which consists in placing a set of linearly arranged transducers (transmitters and receivers) along a plate or hollow cylinder axis (in human body, for example, the diaphysis of long bones). The receivers detect the ultrasound waves that have propagated along the cortical shell, and some parameters can be estimated for tissue characterization. The first AT commercially available device used a 250-kHz pulse transmitted in the mid-tibia cortical layer (Foldes et al., 1995).

9.3. *QUS* Parameters

9.3.1. Transverse Transmission

In transverse transmission, one of the most explored QUS parameter is the **speed of sound (SOS)**, in m/s. Considering the experimental setup from Figure 9.1, the frequency-independent version of SOS can be found using the equation (Laugier, 2008)

$$SOS = \frac{1}{\frac{1}{c_{ref}} + \frac{\Delta TOF}{L}}, \qquad (9.1)$$

where c_{ref} is the ultrasound longitudinal velocity of the reference medium (water is commonly used), ΔTOF is the difference of time-of-flights (TOF) of the reference signal and of the signal transmitted through the sample, and L is the thickness of the measured sample. The frequency-dependent phase velocity $c_p(f)$ can be found in literature (Droin et al., 1998; Laugier, 2008).

Another parameter is the **broadband ultrasonic attenuation (BUA)**. To compute this value, first of all it is necessary to define the apparent frequency-dependent attenuation $\hat{\alpha}(f)L$, using the equation

$$\hat{\alpha}(f)L = \ln\frac{|A_{ref}(f)|}{|A(f)|} \qquad (9.2)$$

where $A_{ref}(f)$ and $A(f)$ are, respectively, the amplitude spectra of the received signal from the reference medium and the analyzed sample. The BUA will be the slope of a linear regression fit to $\hat{\alpha}(f)L$ in the frequency range of 0.2 to 0.6 MHz (Laugier, 2008).

The **backscattering coefficient** $\sigma(f)$ is a QUS parameter mainly used for trabecular bone assessment. It was already presented in Chapter 7, and it can be estimated using the equation

$$\sigma(f) = \frac{1}{V}\left|\frac{k_f^2}{4\pi}\iiint_V [\gamma_\kappa(\vec{r}_o) - \gamma_\rho(\vec{r}_o)] e^{-i\vec{K}\cdot\vec{r}_o} d\vec{r}_o\right|^2, \qquad (9.3)$$

where V is the scattering volume, $k_f = \omega c_f$ (c_f being the acoustic wave velocity in the fluid), γ_κ and γ_ρ are functions which describe the variations in density and compressibility in bone compared to water, respectively; $\vec{K} = -2k_f \hat{z}$ ($\hat{z}$ is the unit vector in the direction of propagation of the incident wave).

More recently in QUS history, the **mean scatterer spacing (MSS)** was proposed (frequently using pulse-echo mode) to characterize the periodicity of biological tissues, including trabecular bone. Some tissues present a quasi-periodic structure (structural periodicity), and the presence of pathologies may alter these patterns. The MSS is used to quantify it. *A priori*, it can be easily estimated using the equation

$$MSS = \frac{SOS}{2f_p}, \qquad (9.4)$$

where f_p is the periodicity-related frequency. The information about this periodic pattern may be recorded in the backscattered signal from the sample. Thus, by calculating the signal power spectrum, a peak will be formed at the frequency related to that regularity (f_p). The hard task is to find the correct frequency, therefore several spectral analysis methods have been proposed with different degrees of success (Landini and Verrazzani, 1990; Varghese and Donohue, 1995; Pereira et al., 2002; Machado et al., 2006; Tang and Abeyratne, 2000; Huang et al., 2008).

9.3.2. Axial Transmission

The axial transmission technique can provide QUS parameters from **guided waves**. The simplest method is to use one emitter and one receiver (Figure 9.3) linearly arranged along the longitudinal axis of the sample. One of the most important signal information to be detected is the **first arriving signal (FAS)**, which is considered the first received signal contribution emerging from noise, with the same period of the excitation signal (Figure 9.4). The **FAS time-of-flight** (TOF$_{FAS}$, in µs) is defined as the time location of the first received signal peak (Bossy et al., 2002). Moreover, the **FAS sound pressure level** (SPL$_{FAS}$, in dB) was proposed by Dodd et al. (2007) in fracture assessment to reflect how much the signal energy is attenuated during its propagation thorough the callus. It can be estimated using the equation

$$SPL = 20\log\frac{A_1}{A_0}, \tag{9.5}$$

where A_1 is the FAS amplitude after its propagation through the sample (callus), and A_0 is the FAS amplitude after its propagation along the reference medium (intact bone, without fracture).

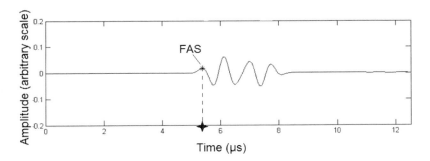

Figure 9.4. The received ultrasound signal after its propagation in axial transmission. The first arriving signal (FAS) can be identified as the first signal contribution.

In more complex devices for axial transmission, probes with more than one emitter/receiver can be used to acquire data: (1) one transmitter-one receiver; (2) one transmitter and several receivers; (3) several transmitters and several receivers' configurations (Talmant et al., 2011). Then different signal processing techniques can be used to extract guided waves velocities. Figure

9.5 shows spatio-temporal signals $r(x,t)$ from an axial transmission device for bidirectional transmission (one emitter at each side of the probe), consisting in a linear array of elements, and a group of fourteen receivers. The FAS velocity can be estimated by calculating the slope of the curve obtained from a linear fit using the position of each FAS.

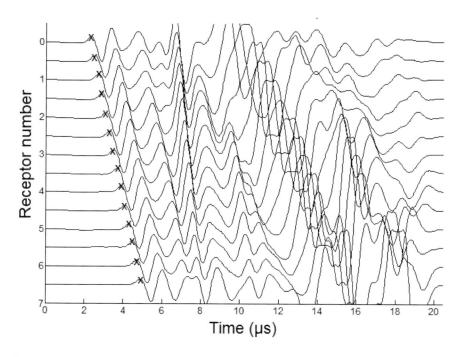

Figure 9.5. Spatio-temporal signals from a bovine intact bone using an multi-element axial transmission device with fourteen receptors. The first arriving signals (FAS) are marked with a "x".

The set of signals $r(x,t)$ shown in Figure 9.5 can be further analyzed in the wavenumber-frequency (k - f) domain. For the general case, the spatio-temporal Fourier transform is given by (Talmant et al., 2011)

$$R(k,f) = \iint_{x,t} r(x,t) e^{-i\omega t} e^{+ikx} dx dt \qquad (9.6)$$

where ω is the angular frequency. This spectral approach has already been applied for fracture healing monitoring, and it will be discussed in the next section.

Some studies have been proposing the use of more sophisticated signal processing techniques for the analysis of the matrix $R(k,f)$, such as the singular value decomposition (SVD), which can provide the guided mode phase velocities using a projection in the singular vector basis. More details are found in other literature (Vrabie et al., 2004; Sasso et al., 2009).

9.4. On the Role of *QUS* in Fracture Healing Assessment: Scientific Evidence

QUS was used for the first time in fracture healing monitoring by the group of Anast et al. (1958). It was an *in vivo* study, in which the ultrasound SOS was measured at different healing stages and compared to contralateral (used as control) intact bones. With a heterogeneous sample (different patients with different healing stages), they observed that SOS returned to 80% of the control value when the patient was able to full weight-bearing.

After this milestone, some studies were presented with different animal models:

- Ultrasound velocity returned on average to 94% of the control value, in completely healed femoral fracture models with guinea pigs (Floriani et al., 1967), using a 100-kHz transducer;
- The modulus of elasticity may have a linear relation to that determined by ultrasound measurements (100 kHz), in mid-femoral models, also with guinea pigs (Abendschein and Hyatt, 1972);
- Using New Zealand white rabbit tibiae, moderate correlations were found between ultrasound measurements (500 kHz and 1 MHz) and physical parameters like load at failure, stiffness and modulus of elasticity. Higher correlations were found for 1-MHz results (perhaps because of the thickness/wavelength ratio - see Chapter 7) (Gill et al., 1989).

Gerlanc et al. (1975) were the first to conduct clinical trials to monitor fracture healing using velocity measurements at 100 kHz. They observed that the severity of fractures may difficult the monitoring with ultrasound. Then in 1996, an important study from Saulgozis et al. (1996) used four 200-kHz transducers for axial transmission measurements to determine SOS and attenuation in fractures. The sample for the *in vivo* approach was composed of subjects without any injury, and patients with tibial fractures (consolidation periods of 1 and 3 weeks). For the *in situ* case, tibiae were used with induced fractures. They have shown that: (1) there was an increase in energy attenuation in the presence of fracture (*in vivo*); (2) bone fractures affected the velocity and the attenuation *in situ*; (3) the overlying soft tissues have not seemed to alter ultrasound measurements; (4) internal fixation may affect ultrasound parameters.

Although its relative simplicity, the work of Lowet and Van der Perre (1996) was significant for the use o QUS in fracture healing evaluation. Indeed they simply measured the SOS with an axial transmission (AT) setup (a 200-kHz transmitter and a receiver) using as a bone-mimicking material (phantom) steel, polyvinylchloride (PVC) and polymethylmetacrylate (PMMA) bars. Figure 9.6 is an illustration of the experimental setup: the transmitter was placed at a fixed position, touching the water surface, and the receiver was moved along the bar axis, in steps of 2 mm. Figure 9.7 shows the results of the wave propagation time (from the transmitter to the receiver) as the distance between the transducer increases, for intact bar, closed gap, 10-mm and 20-mm gap. They have shown that the propagation time increases when the receiver passes above the fracture, and that this time is proportional to the fracture length. Consequently, a hypothesis could be made: ultrasound AT could be a very promising tool for fracture monitoring in long bones in which only a relatively thin soft tissue layer covers its cortical surface.

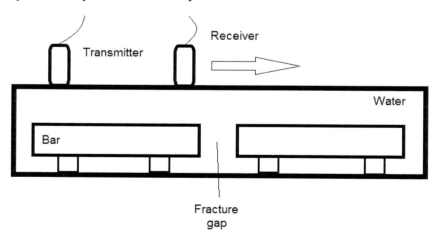

Figure 9.6. Illustration of the experimental setup used by Lowet and Van der Perre (1996) to measure ultrasound propagation time in two bars simulating a fracture. The transmitter was placed at a fixed position, and the receiver was moved along the bar axis (steps of 2 mm).

Almost 10 years later, a group from Greece began their contribution in this field. Malizos et al. (2006) and Protopappas et al. (2005) proposed the application of the transosseous low-intensity pulsed ultrasound (LiUS) on the enhancement and monitoring of fracture healing (a dual approach assessment-therapy). This technique consisted in the implantation of two ultrasound transducers into the fracture site in contact with cortical bone (Figure 9.8), and a wearable platform supporting wireless data communication. The system generated 200-μs bursts of 1-MHz sine waves with an average intensity of 30 mW/cm^2 for a daily 20-minutes treatment, and QUS measurements (TOF$_{FAS}$) could be made in the same device.

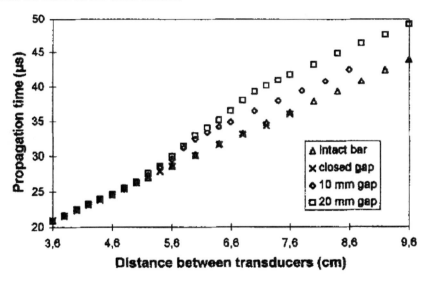

Figure 9.7. Ultrasound propagation time with increasing distance between transducers. Results for intact bar, closed gap, 10-mm and 20-mm gap (Reprinted from Journal of Biomechanics, vol. 29, n. 10, G. Lowet, G. Van der Perre, Ultrasound velocity measurement in long bones: measurement method and simulation of ultrasound wave propagation, p. 1258, Copyright (1996) with permission from Pergamon).

The animal model used was a sheep. In addition, radiographs, destructive three-point bending testing and quantitative computerized tomography to estimate bone mineral density (BMD) were used to correlate callus properties with ultrasound parameters. The authors have demonstrated that wave velocity could be used as a discrimination parameter between healed and nonhealed bones (Figure 9.9), and strong correlations (from 0.69 to 0.81) were found between ultrasound velocity and callus mechanical properties.

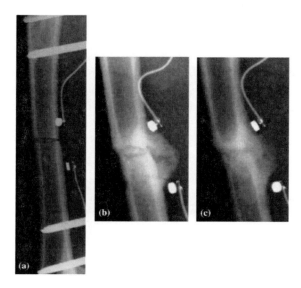

Figure 9.8. X-rays showing the LiUS system, a pair of implantable transducers in contact with bone near the fracture site (sheep as animal model). In (a), a radiograph immediately after the surgical intervention; in (b), after two months; and in (c) before animal sacrifice (Reprinted from Bone, vol. 38, n. 4, Konstantinos Malizos, Athanasios Papachristos, Vasilios Protopappas, Dimitrios Fotiadis, Transosseus application of low-intensity ultrasound for the enhancement and monitoring of fracture healing process in a sheep osteotomy model, p. 532, Copyright (2006) with permission from Elsevier).

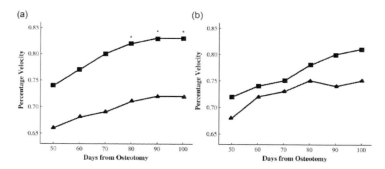

Figure 9.9. Propagation velocity results during the fracture healing process for healed (■) and nonhealed (▲) animals, showing that the velocity was constantly higher for healed fractures. Some significant differences (marked with *) were observed for animals sacrificed 80 days after surgery. (a) and (b) are the results for different observer assessments (Reprinted from Bone, vol. 38, n. 4, Konstantinos Malizos, Athanasios Papachristos, Vasilios Protopappas, Dimitrios Fotiadis, Transosseus application of low-intensity ultrasound for the enhancement and monitoring of fracture healing process in a sheep osteotomy model, p. 536, Copyright (2006) with permission from Elsevier).

In 2006, the same group (Protopappas et al., 2006) studied the propagation of guided waves in intact and healing bones, for the first time by means of two-dimensional (2D) simulations. Simple numerical models were proposed (Figure 9.10) to evaluate FAS velocity measurements during the regeneration process. The transverse fracture gap was 2-mm wide, and the callus consolidation was modeled as a 7-stage process, in which mechanical properties changed as a function of the properties of blood and cortical bone. For axial transmission measurements, they used a transmitter-receiver configuration with two central frequencies tested: 1 MHz and 500 kHz. Moreover, they followed a time-frequency (t-f) signal analysis methodology to evaluate the effect of callus properties and geometry on the dispersion of guided modes, and *ex vivo* experiments were performed on an intact sheep tibia. The FAS corresponded to the lateral wave (Chapter 7), and its velocity increased during the healing stages, but could not be affected by changes in callus geometry. Nevertheless the dispersion of Lamb modes was influenced by both the mechanical and geometrical callus properties. The authors recognized that the Lamb wave approach has some limitations for *in vivo* measurements, because of the presence of soft tissues, inhomogeneity, anisotropy and irregular geometry.

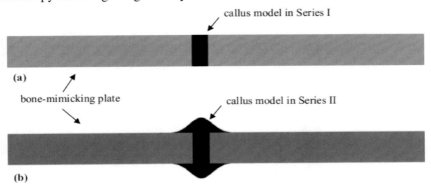

Figure 9.10. Numerical models used for fracture healing monitoring 2D simulations. In (a), there is no callus geometry information; in (b), a periosteal and endosteal callus region is observed(Reprinted from Ultrasound in Medicine & Biology, vol. 32, n. 5, Vasilios Protopappas, Dimitriou Fotiadis, Konstantinos Malizos, Guided ultrasound wave propagation in intact and healing long bones, p. 696, Copyright (2006) with permission from Elsevier).

One year later, they published results from 3D simulations (Protopappas et al., 2007) to better address this issue. The callus is now considered a tissue with several ossification regions (initial connective tissue, soft callus, intermediate stiffness callus, stiff callus and ossified callus) depending on the healing stage (stages 0, 1, 2 and 3), as it can be seen in Figure 9.11. Cortical bone was studied both as an isotropic and transverse isotropic solid. After simulations with an axial transmission configuration (Figure 9.12), they confirmed the fact that FAS was not affected by geometric features (considering comparable dimensions between cortical thickness and ultrasonic wavelength). Higher-order modes of guided waves were sensitive to geometry and anisotropy of bone; however they could not provide quantitative parameters for fracture healing monitoring. Figure 9.13 shows t-f signal representations which demonstrate the sensitivity of guided modes to callus mechanical properties. The properties of the callus tissue from stage 1 to stage 3 significantly influenced the propagation of guided modes. The fundamental modes and the L(0,5) mode at stages 0 and 3 became similar. Guo et al. (2008) commented this work in a letter to the editor, arguing that the t-f representation method alone could not provide monitoring capabilities, and they suggested an association with the normal mode expansion (NME) method or image analysis techniques to better recognize each individual guided mode separately.

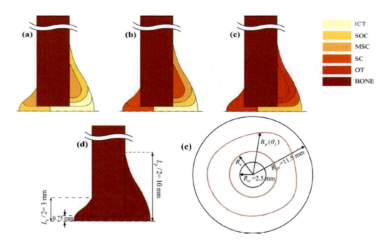

Figure 9.11. Composition of one quarter of the callus tissue for 3D numerical simulations (ICT = initial connective tissue; SOC = soft callus; MSC = intermediate stiffness callus; SC = stiff callus; OT = ossified tissue). Stages 1, 2, 3 and 0 are illustrated in (a), (b), (c) and (d), respectively. In (e), the geometry of the healing bone in a cross-section (Reprinted with permission from The Journal of the Acoustical Society of America, vol. 121, n. 6, Vasilios Protopappas, Iraklis Kourtis, Lampros Kourtis, Konstantinos Malizos, Christos Massalas, Dimitrios Fotiadis, Three-dimensional finite element modeling of guided ultrasound wave propagation in intact and healing long bones, p. 3911, Copyright (2007), Acoustic Society of America).

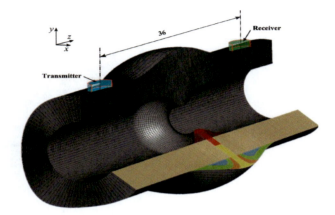

Figure 9.12. 3D simulation setup for axial transmission measurements in fractured bone (Reprinted with permission from The Journal of the Acoustical Society of America, vol. 121, n. 6, Vasilios Protopappas, Iraklis Kourtis, Lampros Kourtis, Konstantinos Malizos, Christos Massalas, Dimitrios Fotiadis, Three-dimensional finite element modeling of guided ultrasound wave propagation in intact and healing long bones, p. 3913, Copyright (2007), Acoustic Society of America).

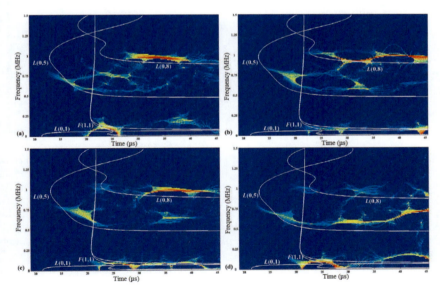

Figure 9.13. T-f representations of the healing bone in (a) stage 0, (b) stage 1, (c) stage 2, and (d) stage 3 (Reprinted with permission from The Journal of the Acoustical Society of America, vol. 121, n. 6, Vasilios Protopappas, Iraklis Kourtis, Lampros Kourtis, Konstantinos Malizos, Christos Massalas, Dimitrios Fotiadis, Three-dimensional finite element modeling of guided ultrasound wave propagation in intact and healing long bones, p. 3919, Copyright (2007), Acoustic Society of America).

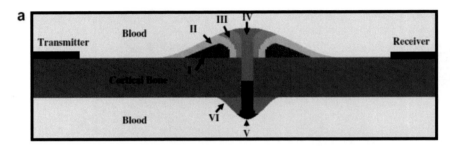
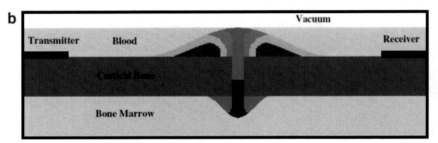
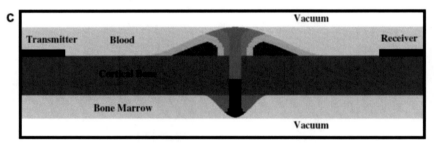

Figure 9.14. Numerical models used in the work of Vavva et al. (2008): (a) bone immersed in blood occupying the semi-infinite spaces (model 1); (b) 2 mm-thick layer of blood on the upper side, and a semi-infinite space of bone marrow on the lower side of the plate (model 2); (c) presence of three layers (model 3) (Reprinted from Ultrasonics, vol. 48, n. 6-7, Maria Vavva, Vasilios Protopappas, Leonidas Gergidis, Antonios Charalambopoulos, Dimitrios Fotiadis, Demos Polyzos, The effect of boundary conditions on guided wave propagation in two-dimensional models of healing bone, p. 602, Copyright (2008) with permission from Elsevier).

Continuing these studies with simulations, Vavva et al. (2008) presented 2D simulations using the commercial software Wave2000 Pro (CyberLogic Inc., NY, USA) to verify the possible effects of the surrounding tissues in a healing bone model on guided wave propagation. They assumed three models, as it can be seen in Figure 9.14, in three stages of healing. The velocity of FAS was measured, and the propagation of guided modes was studied using t-f representations. It was observed that FAS velocity was not affected by fluid boundary conditions (different models). Nevertheless, guided waves were influenced by the overlying soft tissue. Additional modes generated due to the reflections on the free boundary of the blood layer were also found (models 2 and 3). Figure 9.15 shows snapshots from numerical simulations in the healing bone model 2 at stage 2. The transducers are in contact with the cortical bone. It is possible to observe a leakage of waves from the cortical bone into the fluid. In figure 9.15(c), the propagation of waves into callus tissue.

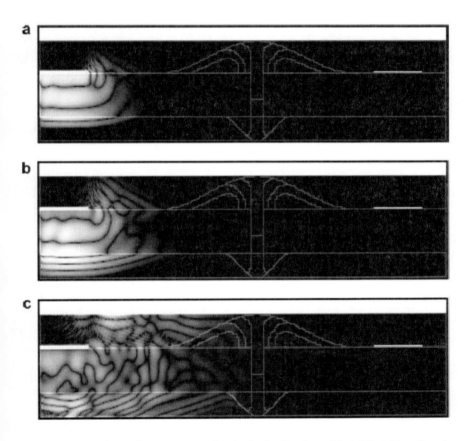

Figure 9.15. Snapshots of wave propagation in the healing bone Model-2 at Stage 2, using commercial software Wave2000 Pro, recorded at (a) 3 μs, (b) 10 μs, and (c) 17 μs (Reprinted from Ultrasonics, vol. 48, n. 6-7, Maria Vavva, Vasilios Protopappas, Leonidas Gergidis, Antonios Charalambopoulos, Dimitrios Fotiadis, Demos Polyzos, The effect of boundary conditions on guided wave propagation in two-dimensional models of healing bone, p. 603, Copyright (2008) with permission from Elsevier).

Other important studies were developed from an English group of researchers. Dodd et al. (2007a) used Sawbones® plates (Pacific Research Laboratories, Inc., USA) and bovine femora to experimentally simulate a transverse fracture. Numerical simulations were also performed with Wave2000 Pro. The measurement configuration is demonstrated in Figure 9.16. The frequency used was 200 kHz. The receiver was moved over a specified distance at 1-mm intervals, and acquired a RF-signal at each position. They measured energy attenuation in axial transmission measurements using the SPL (equation (9.5), in dB). The signal amplitude was sensitive to the presence of small lengths of fractures. When the wave reached the fracture gap, the peak amplitude showed a variation, from which the authors hypothesized that it could be caused by interference between reradiated and scattered/diffracted waves at the fracture site.

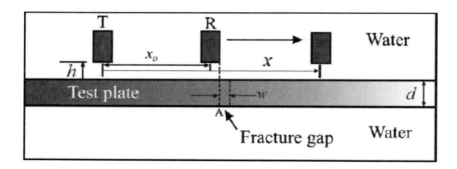

Figure 9.16. Illustration of the axial transmission configuration used by Dodd et al. (2007a). T and R represent the emitter and the receiver, respectively; x_0 is the initial transducer separation, x is the transducer separation, d is the plate thickness, h is the distance between the transducer and the plate, and w is the fracture gap length. The point A under the fracture gap is the starting position of the receiver, and the arrow indicates the direction of receiver motion (Reprinted from Bone, vol. 40, n. 3, S. P. Dodd, J. L. Cunningham, A. W. Miles, S. Gheduzzi, V. F. Humphrey, An *in vitro* study of ultrasound signal loss across simple fractures in cortical bone mimics and bovine cortical bone samples, p. 657, Copyright (2007) with permission from Elsevier).

In Figure 9.17, some important events are worthy of attention:

- In Figure 9.17(a), the lateral wave (re-radiated wave A), propagating from the left to the right, approaches interface 1;
- Figure 9.17(b) shows the scattering or diffraction of wave B, inside fracture gap;

- Consequently, part of the energy from wave B generates a second lateral wave (wave C) in the interface 2, as seen in Figure 9.17(c);
- Since simulations did not account for absorption, the authors stated that FAS attenuation were dependent on two factors: impedance mismatch between bone (plate) and water, and the increase in fracture length.

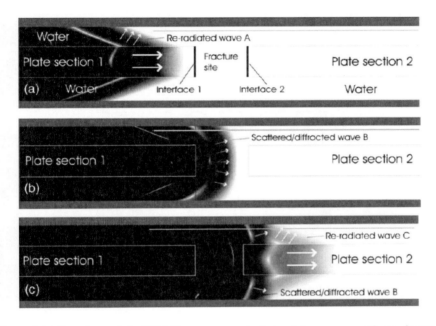

Figure 9.17. Snapshots of the 200-kHz wave numerical simulation across a 10-mm fracture gap. (a), (b) and (c) are three moments of the simulation (Reprinted from Bone, vol. 40, n. 3, S. P. Dodd, J. L. Cunningham, A. W. Miles, S. Gheduzzi, V. F. Humphrey, An *in vitro* study of ultrasound signal loss across simple fractures in cortical bone mimics and bovine cortical bone samples, p. 660, Copyright (2007) with permission from Elsevier).

Further studies from the same group were done. Dodd et al (2007b) simulated different healing stages, with numerical models of a simple and oblique fracture, and a symmetric external callus. A large energy loss in signal amplitude for both transverse and oblique fractures was found. The presence of a callus geometry also reduced wave energy across the fracture. In 2008, using experimental data from bovine femora, they identified an extra time delay compared with the baseline measurement of the intact bone, and this delay increased as the fracture gap widened. A significant loss in signal amplitude relative to the baseline data was observed, at the maximum separation measured, and higher signal loss for oblique fractures. Some results of this paper can be seen in Figures 9.18 and 9.19.

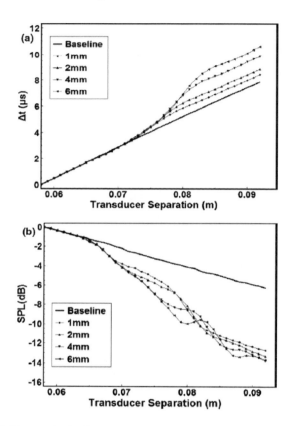

Figure 9.18. (a) Time arrival (Δt) and (b) SPL experimental results from a intact bovine femur (baseline) and transverse fracture of 1, 2, 4 and 6 mm (Reprinted from Ultrasound in Medicine & Biology, vol. 34, n. 3, Simon Dodd, James Cunningham, Anthony Miles, Sabina Gheduzzi, Victor Humphrey, Ultrasound transmission loss across transverse and oblique bone fractures: an *in vitro* study, p. 457, Copyright (2008) with permission from Elsevier).

Moreover, Gheduzzi et al. (2009) developed simulations and an experimental study using Sawbones® plates and bone cement (Palacos® R) to model the cortical bone and the callus, respectively. Figure 9.20 is an illustration of the numerical model used to simulate six stages of healing. Simulations were run using Wave2000® Pro (Figure 9.21). The results corroborated previous findings about FAS velocity and attenuation. Changes in signal amplitude were more evident in the first stages of healing (stages 1 to

2) and in stages 5 to 6 (these two stages being highly dependent on Young's modulus). The addition of a bone cement callus in *in vitro* experiments increased the signal transmission through the fracture gap. When the bone cement was used to mimic the external callus, an increased signal loss was observed compared to just the gap filled alone. These findings suggested that axial transmission could potentially monitor the fracture healing process.

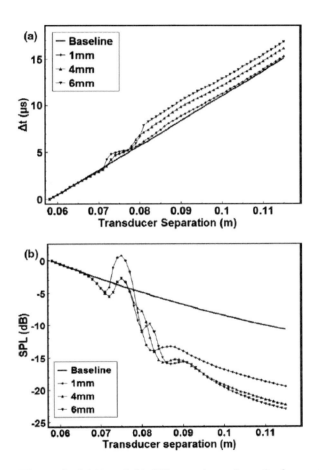

Figure 9.19. (a) Time arrival (Δt) and (b) SPL experimental results from a intact bovine femur (baseline) and oblique (40° to the vertical) fracture of 1, 4 and 6 mm (Reprinted from Ultrasound in Medicine & Biology, vol. 34, n. 3, Simon Dodd, James Cunningham, Anthony Miles, Sabina Gheduzzi, Victor Humphrey, Ultrasound transmission loss across transverse and oblique bone fractures: an *in vitro* study, p. 459, Copyright (2008) with permission from Elsevier).

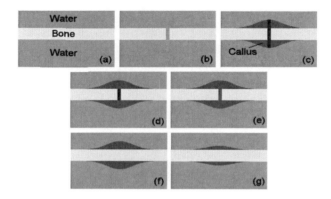

Figure 9.20. Numerical models simulating six stages of healing: (a) intact bone; (b) stage 1: initial fracture; (c) stage 2: the hard callus (dark gray) forms the cartilage bridging (black); (d) stage 3: cartilage remaining only in the fracture gap; (e) stage 4: no cartilage material inside fracture; (f) and (g) stages 5 and 6: callus remodeling (Reprinted with permission from The Journal of the Acoustical Society of America, vol. 126, n. 2, Sabina Gheduzzi, Simon Dodd, Anthony Miles, Victor Humphrey, James Cunningham, Numerical and experimental simulation of the effect of long bone fracture healing stages on ultrasound transmission across an idealized fracture, p. 889, Copyright (2009), Acoustic Society of America).

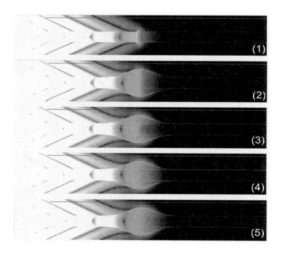

Figure 9.21. Snapshots from numerical simulations for healing stages 1 to 5 (Reprinted with permission from The Journal of the Acoustical Society of America, vol. 126, n. 2, Sabina Gheduzzi, Simon Dodd, Anthony Miles, Victor Humphrey, James Cunningham, Numerical and experimental simulation of the effect of long bone fracture healing stages on ultrasound transmission across an idealized fracture, p. 892, Copyright (2009), Acoustic Society of America).

Researchers from Germany have been publishing interesting results using scanning acoustic microscopy (SAM, see Chapter 6) to evaluate the fracture healing process. Hube et al. (2006) aimed at assessing (using SAM) the mechanical integrity of distracted callus in a sheep model and they compared four clinical treatment concepts for fracture healing: uncoated and coated PDLLA membranes, autologous bone graft surgery from the humerus head, and the association bone graft-membrane. Biomechanical tests were performed to analyze callus mechanical properties. SAM images were obtained by acoustic impedance measurements with a 50-MHz frequency transducer. Figure 9.22 shows examples of SAM images from callus tissue. Using parameters extracted from SAM images, the authors have found a significant linear multivariate regression model to predict the fracture force ($R^2 = 0.86$, p < 0.0001). The best fracture resistance was obtained with the combination of bone graft and coated membrane treatment.

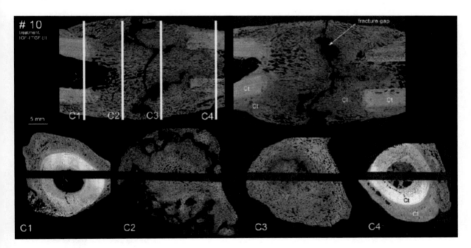

Figure 9.22. Scanning acoustic microscopy (SAM) images from a callus tissue. The upper images are transverse views. Cross-section images are seen in C1 to C4. It is possible to identify the cortical tissue (Ct) and the callus tissue (Cl) (Reprinted from Ultrasound in Medicine & Biology, vol. 32, n. 12, Robert Hube, Hermann Mayr, Werner Hein, Kay Raum, Prediction of biomechanical stability after callus distraction by high resolution scanning acoustic microscopy, p. 1917, Copyright (2006) with permission from Elsevier).

The stiffness, porosity and area of cortical and callus bone tissues with respect to consolidation time and fixator stability were studied by Preininger et al. (2011) in a sheep osteotomy model. The osteotomies were stabilized with either a rigid or a semi-rigid monolateral external fixator attached to the tibia. QUS measurements were performed using SAM to generate high resolution maps of the callus tissue (Figure 9.23). After 2, 3, 6 and 9 weeks postoperative, the animals were sacrificed and the tibiae were biomechanically tested until failure. It was observed that a decrease in cortical stiffness values in regions adjacent to the osteotomy gap during the consolidation period occured (Figure 9.24). For the rigid external fixator group, the stiffness in callus tissue increased from week 3 to week 9.

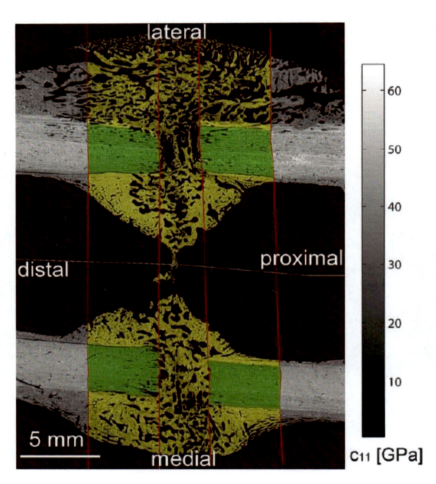

Figure 9.23. High resolution map of a sheep callus using obtained by SAM measurements. The colors indicate segmented regions for analysis (Reprinted from Ultrasound in Medicine & Biology, vol. 37, n. 3, Bernd Preininger, Sara Checa, Ferenc Molnar, Peter Fratzl, Georg Duda, & Kay Raum, Spatial-temporal mapping of bone structural and elastic properties in a sheep model following osteotomy, p. 476, Copyright (2011) with permission from Elsevier).

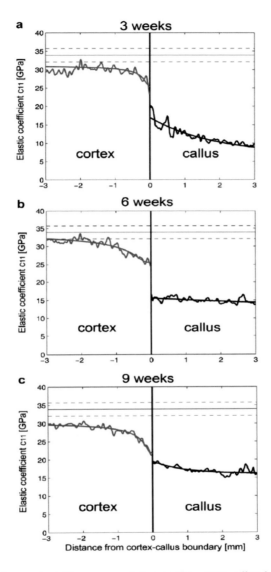

Figure 9.24. Elastic constant C_{11} curves relative to the cortex-callus boundary for (a) 3 weeks; (b) 6 weeks; and (c) 9 weeks of consolidation time. It is possible to identify a smooth elastic transition between cortical bone and periosteal callus in week 9. Mean and standard deviation values for intact bone are depicted by the solid and dashed lines, respectively (Reprinted from Ultrasound in Medicine & Biology, vol. 37, n. 3, Bernd Preininger, Sara Checa, Ferenc Molnar, Peter Fratzl, Georg Duda, & Kay Raum, Spatial-temporal mapping of bone structural and elastic properties in a sheep model following osteotomy, p. 481, Copyright (2011) with permission from Elsevier).

Other interesting approaches of QUS fracture assessment have been proposed by our scientific network Brazil-France. We evaluated the compositional factors in fracture healing affecting axial transmission, using four numerical daily-changing healing models (M1 to M4), representing more realistic clinical conditions, and then verifying the dependence of QUS parameters (TOF$_{FAS}$ and SPL) on callus composition (Machado et al., 2010). Based on finite element simulations by Isaksson et al. (2006), we produced numerical models and used them into a custom-made finite-difference time-domain code named SimSonic2D (Bossy et al., 2004 – www.simsonic.fr) (Figure 9.25 and 9.26). A 1-MHz source and a receiver were positioned parallel to the bone surface to detect the first arriving signal (FAS). TOF$_{FAS}$ was found to be sensitive only to superficial modifications in the propagation path. A stepwise multiple linear regression analysis was performed, showing that callus mature bone alone better explained the variation in TOF$_{FAS}$ ($R^2 \geq 0.70$, $p < 0.001$), and better TOF$_{FAS}$ predictions were obtained when using the callus composition inside cortical fracture gap ($R^2 = 0.98$, $p < 0.01$) (Figure 9.27). The callus composition did not explain the changes in SPL well. Simulations showed that nonunions and delayed unions, as well as the callus degree of mineralization, could be monitored by this technique

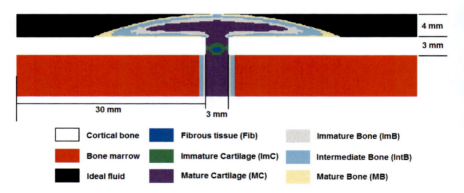

Figure 9.25. Dimensions and tissue composition of the numerical model used for simulations in the study of Machado et al. (2010). The illustration refers to the 6th day of healing from model 1 (Reprinted from Ultrasound in Medicine & Biology, vol. 36, n. 8, Christiano Machado, Wagner Pereira, Maryline Talmant, Frédéric Padilla, Pascal Laugier, Computational evaluation of the compositional factors in fracture healing affecting ultrasound axial transmission measurements, p. 1316, Copyright (2010) with permission from Elsevier).

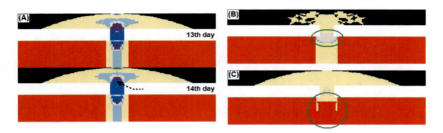

Figure 9.26. Some clinical situations modeled in Machado et al. (2010): (a) 13th and 14th days of bone healing for model 2. The dotted arrow shows an increase in fibrous tissue concentration inside the cortical fracture gap; (b) 100th day of bone healing for model 3, showing an external callus resorption and a nonunion predicted (green circle); (c) 100th day of bone healing for model 4, showing an intramedullary callus resorption (green circle) (Reprinted from Ultrasound in Medicine & Biology, vol. 36, n. 8, Christiano Machado, Wagner Pereira, Maryline Talmant, Frédéric Padilla, Pascal Laugier, Computational evaluation of the compositional factors in fracture healing affecting ultrasound axial transmission measurements, p. 1316, Copyright (2010) with permission from Elsevier).

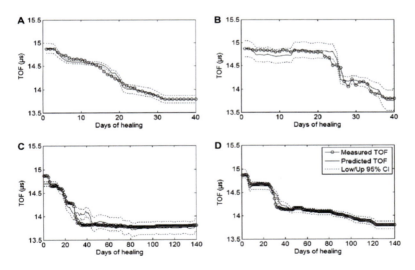

Figure 9.27. Best regression models (dependent variable: TOF$_{FAS}$; independent variables: callus composition): (a) for model 1 (mature bone, intermediate bone and fibrous tissue, $R^2 = 0.98$); (b) for model 2 (mature bone and fibrous tissue, $R^2 = 0.94$); (c) for model 3 (mature, intermediate and immature bone ($R^2 = 0.92$); and (d) for model 4 (mature bone, mature cartilage and fibrous tissue, $R^2 = 0.97$) (Reprinted from Ultrasound in Medicine & Biology, vol. 36, n. 8, Christiano Machado, Wagner Pereira, Maryline Talmant, Frédéric Padilla, Pascal Laugier, Computational evaluation of the compositional factors in fracture healing affecting ultrasound axial transmission measurements, p. 1324, Copyright (2010) with permission from Elsevier).

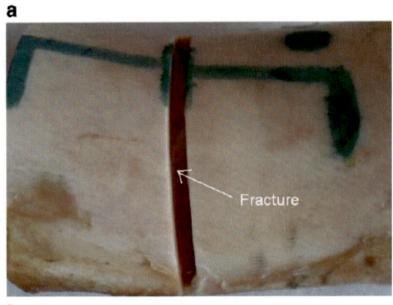

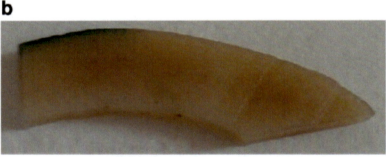

Figure 9.28. (a) The *in vitro* bovine femur sample. It is possible to identify the fracture gap (3 mm). The position of the ultrasound probe for axial transmission is marked. In (b), the cortical bone slice with thickness of 3 mm (Reprinted from Bone, vol. 48, n. 5, Christiano Machado, Wagner Pereira, Mathilde Granke, Maryline Talmant, Frédéric Padilla, Pascal Laugier, Experimental and simulation results on the effect of cortical bone mineralization in ultrasound axial transmission measurements: a model for fracture healing ultrasound monitoring, p. 1203, Copyright (2011) with permission from Elsevier).

One year later, the authors proposed a model for fracture healing monitoring, in an attempt to better document the sensitivity of axial transmission to pure mineralization changes (Machado et al., 2011). They proposed an experimental model in which the degree of mineralization of a bone segment was controlled through a progressive demineralization process. A cortical bovine femur sample was used, in which a 3 mm fracture gap was drilled (Figure 9.28(a)). A 3 mm thick cortical bone slice was extracted from another location in the bone sample (Figure 9.28(b)), and submitted to progressive demineralization process with EDTA (a calcium-specific chelant) during 12 days.

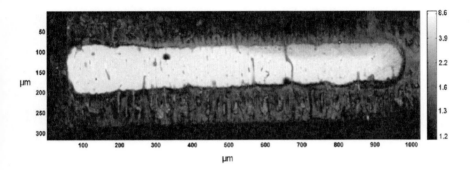

Figure 9.29. Image from scanning acoustic microscopy (50 MHz) of the cortical slice after the demineralization process. It is possible to observe the ossified core (mean impedance = 5.9 ± 0.4 MRayl) and the demineralized region (mean impedance = 1.4 ± 0.1 MRayl) (Reprinted from Bone, vol. 48, n. 5, Christiano Machado, Wagner Pereira, Mathilde Granke, Maryline Talmant, Frédéric Padilla, Pascal Laugier, Experimental and simulation results on the effect of cortical bone mineralization in ultrasound axial transmission measurements: a model for fracture healing ultrasound monitoring, p. 1206, Copyright (2011) with permission from Elsevier).

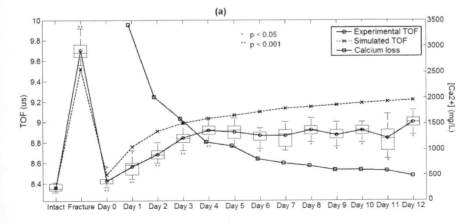

Figure 9.30. (Continued).

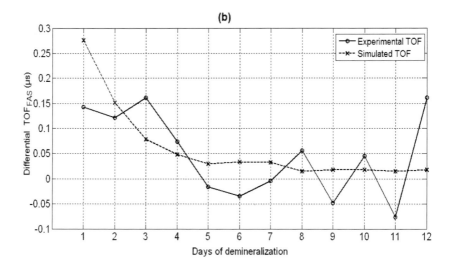

Figure 9.30. In (a), boxplots of the experimental TOF$_{FAS}$ as function of time for the following experimental configuration: before fracture (intact), with fracture gap filled with gel (fracture), with fracture gap filled with the full mineralized bone slice (day 0), with fracture gap filled with the gradually demineralized bone slice (from days 1 to 12). It also depicts the curves for experimental and simulated TOF, as well as calcium loss for each day. In (b), differential experimental and simulated TOF$_{FAS}$ (∂TOF$_{FAS}/\partial t$) obtained from day 1 to day 12 is shown (Reprinted from Bone, vol. 48, n. 5, Christiano Machado, Wagner Pereira, Mathilde Granke, Maryline Talmant, Frédéric Padilla, Pascal Laugier, Experimental and simulation results on the effect of cortical bone mineralization in ultrasound axial transmission measurements: a model for fracture healing ultrasound monitoring, p. 1206, Copyright (2011) with permission from Elsevier).

Axial transmission measurements and simulations were performed using a 1 MHz probe with the demineralized slice placed into the fracture gap to mimic different stages of mineralization. The calcium loss of the slice was recorded and its temporal evolution was modeled by an exponential law. The scanning acoustic microscopy at 50 MHz was also applied to evaluate the mineralization degree of the bone slice at the end of the intervention (Figure 9.29). The authors found a significant and progressive increase in TOF$_{FAS}$ during the beginning of the demineralization process (first 4 days) (Figure 9.30(a)). Simulated and experimental TOF$_{FAS}$ exhibited a similar time-dependence, validating the simulation approach (Figure 9.30(b)). The results showed the dependence between the time-of-flight and local mineralization.

Finally, Rohrbach et al. (2013) reported for the first time the feasibility of transverse transmission quantitative ultrasound in assessment of the onset of cartilage formation during callus formation. They tried to distinguish the early healing phases in a rat osteotomy (OT) model, with a 5-MHz focused transmission system. They imaged the bone repair region after a 2-mm OT, by means of 2-D projection images of speed of sound, time-of-flight and wave attenuation (measured in vitro). The OT gap was assessed by histological analysis and µCT. Fibrous tissue inside the gap was found to have similar properties compared with adjacent muscle tissue, whereas cartilage and mineralized callus tissues differed significantly.

Conclusion

Since the first study in 1958, scientific evidence has demonstrated the possibility of using QUS for fracture healing monitoring and assessment. The delay in time arrival and energy loss of ultrasound during its passage through the fracture gap may be affected by mechanical and geometric properties of the callus tissue. Furthermore, it seems that mineralization plays a key role in these measurements, since it affects the Young's modulus and consequently the speed of sound. During the fracture healing process by secondary ossification, the callus tissue is constantly under mechanical changes. It is widely known that ultrasound is very sensitive to its alterations in the propagation medium, therefore QUS parameters may be a promising tool in this clinical application.

Computer simulations have aided researchers to better evaluate the influence of ultrasound frequency, callus mechanical properties, experimental setups, presence of metallic fixators etc., in the wave propagation. The analysis of a simple lateral wave, or a more complex problem with the Lamb mode, can easily be controlled with specific numerical models coupled with available softwares. For this reason, it seems that numerical approaches may continue to be explored, however with the use of more realistic models from imaging techniques (SAM, µCT).

The interest in ultrasonic fracture healing monitoring as a low-cost, non-ionizing diagnostic tool, mainly using axial transmission techniques, has been growing in the last few decades. Although its increasing development, QUS is still under continuous research and further investigations are needed. Nowadays, unlike in the case of osteoporosis, there is no application in clinical practice, because of the lack of evidence (clinical trials, randomized controlled methodologies, case reports, selection of more homogeneous groups of patients), and are far from clinical acceptance. There is also a need for comparisons between QUS measurements and gold-standard exams like densitometry, computed tomography etc.

The next two chapters will present ultrasound as a therapeutic agent for fracture healing enhancement. In Chapter 10, the bioeffects of ultrasound in biological tissues (specifically during the fracture healing process) will be discussed. The last chapter will deal with the scientific evidences supporting the use of low-intensity pulsed ultrasound to accelerate bone regeneration.

References

Abendschein, W. F., & Hyatt, G. W. (1972). Ultrasonics and physical properties of healing bone. *Journal of Trauma, 12*, 297– 301.

Anast, G. T., Fields, T., & Siegel, I. M. (1958). Ultrasonic technique for the evaluation of bone fractures. *American Journal of Physical Medicine, 37*, 157–159.

Bossy, E., Talmant, M., & Laugier, P. (2002). Effect of bone cortical thickness on velocity measurements using ultrasonic axial transmission: A 2D simulation study. *Journal of the Acoustical Society of America, 112*, 297-307.

Bossy, E., Talmant, M., & Laugier, P. (2004). Three-dimensional simulations of ultrasonic axial transmission velocity measurement on cortical bone models. *The Journal of the Acoustical Society of America, 115*, 2314-2324.

Bossy, E., Laugier, P., Peyrin, F., & Padilla, F. (2007). Attenuation in trabecular bone: A comparison between numerical simulation and experimental results in human femur. *Journal of the Acoustical Society of America, 122*, 2469–2475, 2007.

Dodd, S. P., Cunningham, J. L., Miles, A. W., Gheduzzi, S., & Humphrey, V. F. (2007a). An in vitro study of ultrasound signal loss across simple fractures in cortical bone mimics and bovine cortical bone samples. *Bone, 40*, 656-661.

Dodd, S. P., Miles, A. W., Gheduzzi, S., Humphrey, V. F., & Cunningham, J. L. (2007b). Modelling the effects of different fracture geometries and healing stages on ultrasound signal loss across a long bone fracture. *Computer Methods in Biomechanics and Biomedical Engineering, 10*, 371-375.

Dodd, S. P., Cunningham, J. L., Miles, A. W., Gheduzzi, S., & Humphrey, V. F. (2008). Ultrasound transmission loss across transverse and oblique bone fractures: An *in vitro* study. *Ultrasound in Medicine & Biology, 34*, 454-462.

Droin, P., Berger, G., & Laugier, P. (1998). Dispersion of acoustic waves in cancellous bone. *IEEE Transactions on Ultrasonics, Ferroelectrics, and Frequency Control, 45*, 581-592.

Floriani, L. P., Debervoise, N. T., & Hyatt, G. W. (1967). Mechanical properties of healing bone by use of ultrasound. *Surgical Forum, 18*, 468–470.

Foldes, A. J., Rimon, A., Keinan, D. D., Popovtzer, M. M. (1995). Quantitative ultrasound of the tibia: A novel approach for assessment of bone status. *Bone, 17*, 363-367.

Gerlanc, M., Haddad, D., Hyatt, G. W., Langloh, J. T., & Hilaire, P. S. (1975). Ultrasonic study of normal and fractured bone. *Clinical Orthopaedics and Related Research, 111*, 175–180.

Gheduzzi, S., Dodd, S. P., Miles, A. W., Humphrey, V. F., & Cunningham, J. L. (2009). Numerical and experimental simulation of the effect of long bone fracture healing stages on ultrasound transmission across an idealized fracture. *Journal of Acoustical Society of America, 126*, 887-894.

Gill, P. J., Kernohan, G., Mawhinney, I. N., Mollan, R. A., & McIlhagger, R. (1989). Investigation of the mechanical properties of bone using ultrasound. *Proceedings of the Institution of Mechanical Engineers Part H, 203*, 61–63.

Guo, X., Zhang, D., Yang, D., Gong, X., & Wu, J. (2008). Comment on "Three-dimensional finite element modeling of guided ultrasound wave propagation in intact and healing long bones," [J. Acoust. Soc. Am. 121(6), 3907–3921 (2007)]. *Journal of the Acoustical Society of America, 123*, 4047-4050.

Haïat, G., Padilla, F., & Laugier, P. (2008). Sensitivity of QUS parameters to controlled variations of bone strength assessed with a cellular model. *IEEE Transactions on Ultrasonics, Ferroelectrics, and Frequency Control, 55*, 1488-1496.

Huang, K., Ta, D., Wang, W., & Le, L. H. (2008). Simplified inverse filter tracking algorithm for estimating the mean trabecular bone spacing. *IEEE Transactions on Ultrasonics, Ferroelectrics, and Frequency Control, 55*, 1453-1464.

Hube, R., Mayr, H., Hein, W., & Raum, K. (2006). Prediction of biomechanical stability after callus distraction by high resolution scanning acoustic microscopy. *Ultrasound in Medicine & Biology, 32*, 1913-1921.

Jenson, F., Padilla, F., & Laugier, P. (2003). Prediction of frequency-dependent ultrasonic backscatter in cancellous bone using statistical weak scattering model. *Ultrasound in Medicine & Biology, 29*, 455-464.

Landini, L., & Verrazzani, L. (1990). Spectral characterization of tissue microstructure by ultrasound: a stochastic approach. *IEEE Transactions on Ultrasonics, Ferroelectrics and Frequency Control, 37*, 448-456.

Langton, C. M., Palmer, S. B., & Porter, S. W. (1984). The measurement of broadband ultrasonic attenuation in cancellous bone. *Engineering in Medicine, 13*, 89–91.

Laugier, P. (2008). Instrumentation for in vivo ultrasonic characterization of bone strength. *IEEE Transactions on Ultrasonics, Ferroelectrics, and Frequency Control, 55*, 1179-1196.

Laugier, P. (2011). Quantitative Ultrasound Instrumentation for Bone In Vivo Characterization. In: P. Laugier, & G. Haïat (Eds.), *Bone Quantitative Ultrasound* (1st edition, pp. 47 - 71). New York, NY: Springer.

Litmanovitz, I., Dolfin, T., Friedland, O., Arnon, S., Regev, R., Shainkin-Kestenbaum, R., Lis, M., & Eliakim, A. (2003). Early physical activity intervention prevents decrease of bone strength in very low birth weight infants. *Archives of Disease in Childhood - Fetal and Neonatal Edition, 92*, F381-F385.

Lowet, G., & Van der Perre, G. (1996). Ultrasound velocity measurement in long bones: measurement method and simulation of ultrasound wave propagation. *Journal of Biomechanics, 29*, 1255-1262.

Machado, C. B., Pereira, W. C. A., Meziri, M., & Laugier, P. (2006). Characterization of *in vitro* healthy and pathological human liver tissue periodicity using backscattered ultrasound signals. *Ultrasound in Medicine & Biology, 32*, 649-657.

Machado, C. B., Pereira, W. C. A., Talmant, M., Padilla, F., & Laugier, P. (2010). Computational evaluation of the compositional factors in fracture healing affecting ultrasound axial transmission measurements. *Ultrasound in Medicine & Biology, 36*, 1314-1326.

Machado, C. B., Pereira, W. C. A., Granke, M., Talmant, M., Padilla, F., & Laugier, P. (2011). Experimental and simulation results on the effect of cortical bone mineralization in ultrasound axial transmission measurements: A model for fracture healing ultrasound monitoring. *Bone, 48*, 1202-1209.

Malizos, K. N., Papachristos, A. A., Protopappas, V. C., & Fotiadis, D. I. (2006). Transosseous application of low-intensity ultrasound for the enhancement and monitoring of fracture healing process in a sheep osteotomy model. *Bone, 38*, 530–539.

Marin, F., Gonzalez-Macias, J., Diez-Perez, A., Palma, S., & Delgado-Rodriguez, M. (2006). Relationship between bone quantitative ultrasound and fractures: A meta-analysis. *Journal of Bone and Mineral Research, 21,* 1126–1135.

Pereira, W. C. A., Abdelwahab, A., Bridal, S. L., & Laugier, P. (2002). Singular spectrum analysis applied to 20 MHz backscattered ultrasound signals from periodic and quasi-periodic phantoms. *Acoustical Imaging, 26*, 239-246.

Pereira, W. C. A., Machado, C. B., Negreira, C. A., & Canetti, R. (2008). Ultrasonic Techniques for Medical Imaging and Tissue Characterization. In: A. Arnau (Ed.), *Piezoelectric Transducers and Applications* (2nd edition, pp. 433 - 465). Berlin: Springer-Verlag.

Preininger, B., Checa, S., Molnar, F. L., Fratzl, P., Duda, G. N., & Raum, K. (2011). Spatial-temporal mapping of bone structural and elastic properties in a sheep model following osteotomy. *Ultrasound in Medicine & Biology, 37*, 474-483.

Protopappas, V. C., Baga, D. A., Fotiadis, D., Likas, A. C., Papachristos, A. A., & Malizos, K. N. (2005). An ultrasound wearable system for the monitoring and acceleration of fracture healing in long bones. *IEEE Transactions on Biomedical Engineering, 52,* 1597–1608.

Protopappas, V. C., Fotiadis, D. I., & Malizos, K. N. (2006). Guided ultrasound wave propagation in intact and healing long bones. *Ultrasound Medicine & Biology, 32*, 693-708.

Protopappas, V. C., Kourtis, I. C., Kourtis, L., C., Malizos, K. N., Massalas, C. V., & Fotiadis, D. I. (2007). Three-dimensional finite element modeling of guided ultrasound wave propagation in intact and healing long bones. *Journal of the Acoustical Society of America, 121*, 3907-3921.

Rohrbach, D., Preininger, B., Hesse, B., Gerigk, H., Perka, C., & Raum, K. (2013). The early phases of bone healing can be differentiated in a rat osteotomy model by focused transverse-transmission ultrasound. *Ultrasound in Medicine & Biology, 39*, 1642-1653.

Saulgozis, J., Pontaga, I., Lowet, G., & Van der Perre, G. (1996). The effect of fracture and fracture fixation on ultrasonic velocity and attenuation. *Physiological Measurement, 17*, 201–211.

Sasso, M., Talmant, M., Haïat, G., Naili, S., & Laugier, P. (2009). Analysis of the most energetic late arrival in axially transmitted signals in cortical bone. *IEEE Transactions on Ultrasonics, Ferroelectrics and Frequency Control, 56*, 2463-2470.

Siegel, I. M., Anast, G. T., & Fields, T. (1958). The determination of fracture healing by measurement of sound velocity across the fracture site. *Surgery, Gynecology & Obstetrics, 107*, 327–332.

Talmant, M., Foiret, J., Minonzio, J.-G. (2011). Guided Waves in Cortical Bone. In: P. Laugier, & G. Haïat (Eds.), *Bone Quantitative Ultrasound* (1st edition, pp. 147 - 179). New York, NY: Springer.

Tang, X., & Abeyratne, U. R. (2000). Wavelet transforms in estimating scatterer spacing from ultrasound echoes. *Ultrasonics, 38*, 688-692.

Varghese, T., & Donohue, K. D. (1995). Estimating mean scatterer spacing with the frequency-smoothed spectral autocorrelation function. *IEEE Transactions on Ultrasonics, Ferroelectrics and Frequency Control, 42*, 451-463.

Vavva, M. G., Protopappas, V. C., Gergidis, L. N., Charalambopoulos, A., Fotiadis, D., & Polyzos, D. (2008). The effect of boundary conditions on guided wave propagation in two-dimensional models of healing bone. *Ultrasonics, 48*, 598-606.

Vrabie, V. D., Mars, J. I., & Lacoume, J. L. (2004). Modified singular value decomposition by means of independent component analysis. *Signal Processing, 84*, 645-652.

Wear, K. (2008). A method for improved standardization of *in Vivo* Calcaneal Time-Domain Speed-of-Sound Measurements. *IEEE Transactions on Ultrasonics, Ferroelectrics, and Frequency Control, 55*, 1473-1479.

Section IV - Ultrasound as a Therapeutic Tool for Fracture Healing

Chapter 10

Bioeffects of Ultrasound in Fracture Regeneration

Abstract

Both therapeutic and diagnostic ultrasound may lead to various effects in biological tissue. These effects can be classified into two categories: thermal (temperature elevation induced by the passage of ultrasound waves through the tissue) and nonthermal or mechanical effects (contributing only with a mechanical stimulation). There are three main mechanisms for the generation of thermal effects: heat conduction, absorption and perfusion. Nonthermal effects are represented by cavitation (formation of tiny gas bubbles in the tissues caused by ultrasound stimulation), and acoustic streaming, divided into two categories: the bulk streaming (fluid moving in a single direction) and microstreaming (formation of eddies of flow). The applications of therapeutic ultrasound can be, amongst others, soft tissue stimulation, bone regeneration, cancer therapy, stimulation of immune response and hemostasis, as well as specific biomolecular effects (alterations in membrane permeability, increase in intracellular calcium concentration, activation of ion channels and gene transfection). The enhancement of fracture healing using low-intensity pulsed ultrasound stimulation (LIPUS) has been extensively researched in the last decades, and some hypothesis for probable causes were already developed: mechanical signal transduction and induction of gene expression, activation of enzymes in response to thermal effects, angiogenesis at the fracture site, modulation of intracellular calcium signaling, and enhancement of cartilage calcification and maturation.

10.1. Introduction

As the use of ultrasound in Medicine has become more popular in the last decades, concerns about its bioeffects and patient safety have arisen from scientists worldwide. Nowadays a lot about ultrasound-induced bioeffects is known, although some therapeutic applications (mainly in musculoskeletal rehabilitation by physical therapists) are based on the slogan "if there is no therapeutic effect, at least no harm done", i.e. if the effects of ultrasound in the body are not known, low intensities during a short period of time are permitted to guarantee no harmful consequences to the tissue. Both therapeutic and diagnostic ultrasound may lead to various effects in biological tissue, depending on factors like intensity, frequency, wave generation (pulsed, continuous), tissue impedance, time of application etc. These effects can be classified into two categories: thermal and nonthermal (or mechanical) effects. Thermal effects encompass all phenomena which cause a rise in temperature induced by the passage of ultrasound waves through the body. Nonthermal effects do not provoke *a priori* a significant tissue heating, contributing only with a mechanical stimulation (since ultrasound is the propagation of a mechanical disturbance in a medium). Heating is intensity dependent, and it can be controlled by pulsing the beam (reducing heating) or generating a continuous ultrasound beam (increasing heating).

Physical therapists commonly use the therapeutic ultrasound for long and short-term clinical benefits, mainly in the United States. Nevertheless, whether ultrasound is therapeutically effective or not still requires further investigation, because many applications are supported by empirical conclusions (Feril et al., 2008a). The main objective of this chapter is to present an overview of ultrasound-induced effects in biological tissues (thermal and nonthermal), specifically the influence of acoustic stimulation in fracture gaps and callus to accelerate bone regeneration.

10.2. Ultrasound-Induced Effects in Biological Tissues

10.2.1. Thermal Effects

Ultrasound stimulation in biological tissue provokes a rise in local temperature, which can lead to changes in cellular activity. For example, temperatures from 44 to 46 °C can lead to coagulation of proteins.

Temperatures higher than 45°C denature enzymes, which are specialized proteins for chemical reactions catalysis. An empirical relation was developed by Miller and Ziskin (1989) to estimate the shortest duration t_{exp} for any temperature to cause a detrimental effect. It can be given by

$$t_{exp} = 4^{43-T}, \qquad (10.1)$$

where T is the temperature in °C. One can conclude that the shorter the time for an ultrasound exam or therapeutic application, the smaller the chances for detrimental effects caused by the thermal stimulation.

But how can ultrasound increase tissue temperature during stimulation? According to Szabo (2004), three main effects may be crucial: heat conduction, absorption and perfusion. **Heat conduction** refers to the transducer as a direct source of heat for the body. Self-heating can occur with transducers which are left unused with a high acoustic power, due to the high impedance mismatch between the transducer face and the air. The generated waves are then reflected back, increasing the temperature in the probe.

During ultrasound propagation, the energy is lost to **absorption**, i.e. energy is converted to heat. The pattern of heating is related to the distribution of intensity in the absorbed beam, using the equation (Szabo, 2004)

$$q_{vol} = 2\alpha I \qquad (10.2)$$

where q_{vol} is the volume rate of heat generation, I is the acoustic intensity and α is the absorption coefficient.

Blood **perfusion** is another event which alters tissue temperature during ultrasound stimulation, and it is extremely important for temperature estimation. It was already proven that the temperature may decay exponentially when an uniform temperature distribution is established and the acoustic source is withdrawn, following the equation

$$T = T_0 e^{-t/\tau} \qquad (10.3)$$

where τ is the perfusion time constant. Each tissue presents its own perfusion values.

10.2.2. Nonthermal (Mechanical) Effects

One of the nonthermal effects of ultrasound in biological tissues is cavitation, the behavior of bubbles within an acoustic field. As defined by Low and Reed (1994), cavitation is the formation of tiny gas bubbles in tissues caused by ultrasound stimulation. Acoustic streaming is another mechanical effect, which is divided into two categories: the bulk streaming (when the beam propagates in a liquid, with the fluid moving in a single direction) and microstreaming (formation of eddies of flow adjacent to the oscillating source).

Microstreaming does not occur in vivo, because it should always be associated with cavitation (Baker et al., 2001). Therefore, it is not possible to state that microstreaming induced by ultrasound alter membrane permeability or stimulate cell activity. Other mechanical effects may create particle oscillations, and then lead to mechanical effects (depending on the acoustic intensity).

Other authors have been presenting controversial results about blood cell stasis by stationary waves (Dyson, 1987) and angiogenesis (growth of new blood vessels) (Rubin et al., 1990; Hanahan and Folkman, 1996). It seems that it cannot be reproduced for in vivo conditions.

10.2.3. Therapeutic Applications of Ultrasound

According to a literature review by Paliwal and Mitragotri (2008), some ultrasound therapeutic applications stand out:

- **Soft tissue stimulation**: through its thermal and nonthermal effects. Some findings are (1) the increased extensibility of collagen-rich scar tissues, tendons and joints; (2) pain and muscular spasm relief; (3) cell stimulation cells by upregulation of signaling molecules; (4) activation of immune cells to migrate to the site of injury; (5) wound contraction and scar tissue remodeling;
- **Bone regeneration**: it is widely known that low-intensity ultrasound stimulation ultrasounds enhance the fracture healing mechanism. It is the main theme of this book, and it will be discussed soon in this chapter;

- **Cancer therapy**: ultrasound can present harmful and potentially lethal biological effects which can be used for tumor suppression or elimination. Some applications are: (1) ultrasound-induced microtubule disassembly; (2) ultrasound-induced non-necrotic and localized hyperthermia in tumor tissues (prostate, liver, breast, kidney, sarcoma, and uterus; (3) selective ultrasound induced cellular toxicity in tumor cells.
- **Stimulation of immune response**: ultrasound may increase the efficacy of transcutaneous immunization (application of vaccines on the skin). One of the hypothesis is that acoustic cavitation may breach the skin's barrier resulting in an inflame-matory response needed for the immunization (sonopermea-bilization). Ultrasound also can have a role in the disruption of nanoparticles filled with a specific drug (targeted delivery);
- **Hemostasis:** is the opposite of hemorrhage, i.e. it is a process which causes bleeding to stop. High-intensity focused ultrasound (HIFU) can be employed at 1 to 5 MHz and high intensity (1 to 10 kW/cm^2), focused on the ruptured vasculature, then leading to a necrosis by coagulation and consequent hemostasis.

Therapeutic ultrasound has also been proposed for specific biomolecular effects, and some of these were presented by Feril et al. (2008b):

- Alterations in membrane permeability, cellular adhesion and proliferation, by activating signal transduction pathways that lead to gene regulation;
- Increase in intracellular calcium ion concentration, by changes in membrane mechanisms for ion diffusion;
- Activation of ion channels, membrane proteins, signaling molecules, growth factor membrane receptors, cytoskeletal fila-ments, nuclei, extracellular matrix, and other structures, affecting cellular mechanotransduction;
- Gene transfection (delivery of genes into cells) by ultrasound sonotransfection). The acoustic waves (generally at frequencies lower than 1 MHz) may increase DNA uptake by cells. The possible mechanism iscavitation, but other hypotheses are an escape from endosomes, gene upregulation, alteration of intracellular molecular trafficking, protein translation or creating membrane pores.

10.3. How Can Ultrasound Accelerate Fracture Healing?

The enhancement of fracture healing using low-intensity pulsed ultrasound stimulation (known as LIPUS) has been extensively investigated in the last decades, with tens of review papers recently published (some examples are the reviews from Bashardoust et al., 2012; Albornoz et al., 2011; Gleiza et al., 2011; Watanabe et al., 2010 and Siska et al., 2008). We can observe that the conclusions are always the same: although it is well established that ultrasound can accelerate bone regeneration, the mechanisms underlying this phenomenon are unknown, and further studies are needed. As a consequence only scientific speculations have been proposed.

Siska et al. (2008) presented five potential mechanisms that may be present during an ultrasound stimulation for fracture healing: mechanical signal transduction and induction of gene expression, activation of enzymes in response to thermal effects, angiogenesis at the fracture site, modulation of intracellular calcium signaling, and enhancement of cartilage calcification and maturation.

The cells in our body can be sensitive to several physical stimuli to transduce signals for biological adjustments. Since ultrasound is a mechanical vibration propagated through a medium, the pressure waves can adjunctly act to accelerate the biochemical pathways in bone cells by changing the cellular response, modulating cell function and therefore stimulating the regeneration process (Siska et al., 2008).

Bone and muscle (or bone and hematoma/soft callus) form an interface of high impedance mismatch which lead most of the incident radiation to reflect. Since a fracture is a condition where bone and other lower-impedance structures are present, several reflections are expected inside the discontinuity, resulting in significant acoustic pressure variations through the tissue (Figure 10.1), therefore increasing cellular mechanical stimulation. It is also known that air may also be present in the fracture region after a traumatic injury. In this case, cavitation may be produced by ultrasound stimulation, increasing mechanical stimulation (Hadjiargyrou et al., 1998).

The formation and stability of a callus may also be enhanced because of the induction of gene expression caused by LIPUS. Table 10.1 depicts some of the genes expressed in response to ultrasound stimulation. According to Siska et al. (2008), LIPUS may also modify the activity of gene products in the fracture sites, by for example activating some important enzymes by slight increases of temperature ($< 1°C$).

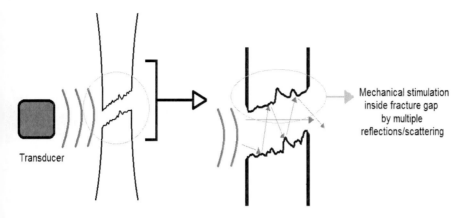

Figure 10.1. The fracture gap is a condition composed by bone and other lower-impedance structures. This high impedance mismatch causes several reflections inside the discontinuity, resulting in significant acoustic pressure variations through the tissue, consequently enhancing mechanical signal transduction.

Table 10.1. Genes expressed and their functions in response to ultrasound stimulation (LIPUS) (Reprinted from Injury, vol. 39, Peter Siska, Gary Gruen, Hans Pape, External adjuncts to enhance fracture healing: What is the role of ultrasound?, p. 1098, Copyright (2008) with permission from Elsevier)

Gene	Function
Aggrecan	Constituent of cartilage
Osteopontin and osteocalcin	Non-collagenous proteins found in bone
Major histocompatibility Class I antigen	Immunologic pathways
Cyr61	Growth factor involved in chondrogenesis
Phosphoglucomutase	Glycolitic enzyme
c-fos	Immediate early gene
Insulin growth factor (IGF-1)	Anabolic gene

Others have showed that LIPUS may stimulate osteogenesis through calcium signaling and consequent cartilage calcification by increasing the levels of intracellular calcium incorporation in cultures of differentiating bone and cartilage cells and enhancing endochondral ossification (Parvizi et al., 2002; Korstjens et al., 2004).

An article published in 2010 in the journal *Medical Hypothesis* (Zhao and Yan, 2010) brought out some questions about the efficacy of LIPUS in fracture healing. The authors hypothesized that LIPUS may increase the concentration of oxygen radicals secreted by neutrophils in healthy osteogenic cells, which could affect the viability of these cells at the acute phase of a fracture (within 1 week). At the same time that neutrophils migrate to the site of inflammation, offering a defense against pathogens or eliminating dead cells, they can release reactive oxygen radicals and proteases, which are very harmful in high intracellular concentrations.

Conclusion

LIPUS is a very attractive tool for the therapeutic management of bone fractures. First of all, it is apparently harmless (despite some hypothesis lately proposed). Secondly, it is simple to use and has a relatively low cost. Ultrasound stimulation can be very useful for specific conditions like comminuted and/or open fractures, associated comorbidities, elderly, smokers and malnutrition. The reduction of the healing time can prevent delayed unions or nonunions, producing cost savings, decrease in disability and a rapid return to prior levels of function in activities of daily living (ADL's).

The application of ultrasound stimulates cells and tissues leading to various mechano-biochemical responses which are of utmost importance for technological health innovations in bioengineering, bone and soft tissue healing, cancer therapy and gene delivery, among others. Nevertheless the mechanisms underlying this therapeutic approach still need further investigation, as the results reported in literature present inconsistencies (lack of controlled randomized trials in humans, different ultrasound parameters etc.).

This chapter provided a brief background about how ultrasound can act as an accelerator of bone regeneration. The next (and last) chapter of this book will present some scientific evidence of the therapeutic application of ultrasound for the enhancement of fracture healing. From *in vitro* to *in vivo* studies, from animal models to human clinical trials, the most important findings will be discussed.

References

Albornoz, P. M., Khanna, A., Longo, U. G., Forriol, F., & Maffuli, N. (2011). The evidence of low-intensity pulsed ultrasound for in vitro, animal and human fracture healing. *British Medical Bulletin, 100*, 39-57.

Bashardoust, T. S., Houghton, P., MacDermid, J. C., & Grewal, R. (2012). Effects of low-intensity pulsed ultrasound therapy on fracture healing. A systematic review and meta-analysis. *American Journal of Physical Medicine and Rehabilitation, 91*, 349-367.

Baker, K. G., Robertson, V. J., & Duck, F. A. (2001). A review of therapeutic ultrasound: biophysical effects. *Physical Therapy, 81*, 1351-1358.

Dyson, M. (1987). Mechanisms involved in therapeutic ultrasound. *Physiotherapy, 73*, 116–120.

Feril, L. B., Tachibana, K., Ogawa, K., Yamaguchi, K., Solano, I. G., & Irie, Y. (2008a). Therapeutic potential of low-intensity ultrasound (part 1): thermal and sonomechanical effects. *Journal of Medical Ultrasonics, 35*, 153-160.

Feril, L. B., Tachibana, K., Ikeda-Dantsuji, Y., Endo, H., Harada, Y., Kondo, T., Ogawa, R. (2008b). Therapeutic potential of low-intensity ultrasound (part 2): biomolecular effects, sonotransfection, and sonopermeabilization. *Journal of Medical Ultrasonics, 35*, 161-167.

Gleizal, A., Lavandier, B., Paris, M., & Béra, J.-C. (2011). Intérêt des ultrasons pulsés de faible intensité dans la stimulation de la régénération osseuse. *Revue de Stomatologie et de Chirurgie Maxillo-faciale, 112*, 233-239.

Hadjiargyrou, M., McLeod, K., Ryaby, J. P., & Rubin, C. (1998). Enhancement of fracture healing by low intensity ultrasound. *Clinical Orthopaedics and Related Research, 355S*, S216-S229.

Hanahan, D., & Folkman, J. (1996). Patterns and emerging mechanisms of the angiogenic switch during tumorigenesis. *Cell, 86*, 353–364.

Korstjens, C. M., Nolte, P. A., Burger, E. H., Albers, G. H., Semeins, C. M., Aartman, I. H., Goei, S. W., & Klein-Nulend, J. (2004). Stimulation of bone cell differentiation by low-intensity ultrasound - a histomorphometric in vitro study. *Journal of Orthopaedical Research, 22*, 495—500.

Low, J., & Reed, A. (1994). *Electrotherapy Explained: Principles and Practice*. Oxford: Butterworth Heinemann.

Miller, M. W., & Ziskin, M. C. (1989). Biological consequences of hyperthermia. *Ultrasound in Medicine & Biology, 26*, 441-450.

Paliwal, S., & Mitragotri, S. (2008). Therapeutic opportunities in biological responses of ultrasound. *Ultrasonics, 48*, 271-278.

Parvizi, J., Parpura, V., Greenleaf, J. F., & Bolander, M. E. (2002). Calcium signaling is required for ultrasound-stimulated aggrecan synthesis by rat chondrocytes. *Journal of Orthopaedical Research, 20*, 51-57.

Rubin, M. J., Etchison, M. R., Condra, K. A., Franklin Jr., T. D., & Snoddy, A. M. (1990). Acute effects of ultrasound on skeletal muscle oxygen tension, blood flow, and capillary density. *Ultrasound in Medicine & Biology, 16*, 271–277.

Siska, P. A., Gruen, G. S., & Pape, H. C. (2008). External adjuncts to enhance fracture healing: what is the role of ultrasound? *Injury, 39*, 1095-1105.

Szabo, T. L. (2004). *Diagnostic Ultrasound Imaging: Inside Out* (1st edition). Burlington: Elsevier Academic Press.

Watanabe, Y., Matsushita, T., Bhandari, M., Zdero, R., & Schemitsch, E. H. (2010). Ultrasound for fracture healing: current evidence. *Journal of Orthopaedical Trauma, 24*, S56-S61.

Zhao, X., & Yan, S.-G. (2011). Low-intensity pulsed ultrasound (LIPUS) therapy may enhance the negative effects of oxygen radicals in the acute phase of fracture. *Medical Hypothesis, 76*, 283-285.

Chapter 11

Therapeutic Ultrasound in Fractures: State of the Art

Abstract

Despite the scientific evidence corroborating the use of ultrasound to enhance fracture healing, the mechanisms underlying this phenomenon are still to be determined. In vitro evidence show that LIPUS may stimulate osteoblastic production of inflammatory mediators and the expression of specific genes. Animal models (rat, sheep, pig, horse) have given important insight about the efficacy of LIPUS. Average intensities of 30 mW/cm^2 SATA, together with frequencies around 1.5 MHz, have been applied with success in most of the studies. On the other hand, several systematic reviews and meta-analysis have been published in the last years presenting successful human clinical (including randomized controlled) trials, involving fresh fractures, delayed or nonunions, and distraction osteogenesis.

11.1. Introduction

It is already well established that ultrasound enhances fracture healing. As seen in Chapter 10, despite the scientific evidence corroborating this therapeutic application, the mechanisms underlying this stimulation are still to be determined. Meanwhile, the possible rationale of this biophysical phenomenon may be the mechanical signal transduction, the induction of gene expression, the activation of enzymes, angiogenesis, intracelullar signaling, and/or the enhancement of cartilage maturation.

Talaji et al. (2012) wrote about first reports of the application of LIPUS in bone regeneration. An osteogenic stimulation using ultrasound was made by Maintz, in 1950, who verified the formation of new periosteal bone a radius osteotomy in rabbits. Corradi and Cozzolino (1953) presented a first clinical trial reporting an enhancement in periosteal callus formation.

An important paper was written by a Brazilian researcher named Luiz Romaris Duarte (1983), in which he described an experiment with 45 rabbits using two models: (1) a bilateral osteotomy of fibula; and (2) bilateral drilled holes on the femur. A daily 15-minutes pulsed ultrasound stimulation was done, with low acoustic intensity, demonstrating that treated animals could have an acceleration in bone regeneration compared to untreated ones. In the same year, Dyson and Brookes (1983) verified this effect of ultrasound in complete bilateral transverse fibular fractures in Wistar rats. A few years later, North American researchers John Peter Ryaby e Roger Talish created the Exogen, a company to manufacture a LIPUS (low-intensity pulsed ultrasound stimulation) unit, which obtained the right to use this technology by the FDA in 1994. In 2001, the British company Smith & Nephew purchased Exogen. Publications in this field became more numerous since 1990.

In the last chapter of this book, some of the most important studies regarding the ultrasound stimulation of fractures will be presented and discussed according to each approach: *in vitro*, animal models and clinical human trials.

11.2. *In Vitro*

In 1998, a systematic review was published by Hadjiargyrou et al., who summarized some of the first evidences for the effect of ultrasound stimulation *in vitro* on fracture healing. Chapman et al. (1980) used acoustic intensities from 0.5 to 3 W/cm^2 (SATA - spatial average temporal average) in thymocytes. They verified a decrease in potassium ion (K^+) content, and at 2 W/cm^2 there was a decrease in K^+ uptake together with an increase of K^+ efflux. Ryaby et al. (1992) observed an increase in adenylate cyclase and transforming growth factor (TGF-β) production in osteoblastic cell lines with ultrasound stimulation at 20 - 45 mW/cm^2. Wu et al. (1996) and Parvizi et al. (1997) found stimulatory effects in chondrocytes (increase in aggrecan mRNA and intracellular calcium release).

Reher et al. (1997) developed a controlled study to assess the effects of different ultrasound intensities on a 5-day-old *in vitro* mouses' calvaria bone. They used an ultrasound unit at 3 MHz, pulsed 1:4, and intensities from 0.1 to 2.0 W/cm^2 SATA. The control group was treated with the device switched off. Collagen and noncollagenous protein synthesis and temperature change were measured. The synthesis of bone matrix proteins was stimulated significantly at 0.1 W/cm^2 (Figure 11.1) and at higher frequencies this synthesis was suppressed (only significant at 2.0 W/cm^2). The authors observed that the mechanical effects were responsible for this response, because the increase in temperature during experiments ranged from 1.8 to 2.0 °C (with no increase in temperature for the experiment at 0.1 W/cm^2).

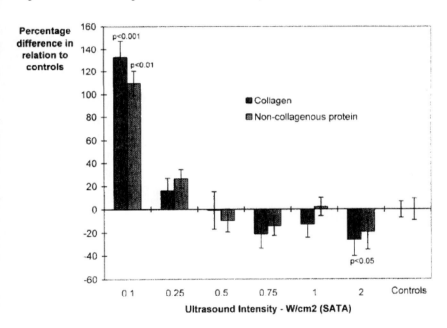

Figure 11.1. Percentage difference of collagen and non-collagenous protein formation in relation to controls, for several ultrasound intensities (Reprinted from Ultrasound in Medicine & Biology, vol. 23, n. 8, Peter Reher, El-Noor Elbeshir, Wilson Harvey, Sajeda Meghji, Malcolm Harris, The stimulation of bone formation in vitro by therapeutic ultrasound, p. 1255, Copyright (1997) with permission from Elsevier).

Doan et al. (1999) and Reher et al. (1999) evaluated *in vitro* effects of ultrasound on cell proliferation, cytokine production and protein synthesis by human fibroblasts, osteoblasts and monocytes, with a 1-MHz pulsed unit and a 45-kHz machine (long waves), at various intensities. Assays were performed for DNA synthesis (cell proliferation), collagen and noncollagenous (NCP) protein synthesis, and ELISA (Enzyme-linked immunosorbent assay) to assess cytokine production (interleukins - IL, tumor necrosis factor α - TNFα, basic fibroblast growth factor - bFGF, and vascular endothelial growth factor - VEGF). The two types of equipment increased cell proliferation between 35% and 52%. Best results for collagen and NCP protein were obtained with a frequency of 45 kHz. It was also observed that ultrasound may stimulate the production of cytokines with both frequencies (Figure 11.2). The optimum intensities were 15 and 30 mW/cm^2 (SATA) for 45 kHz, and 0.1 and 0.4 W/cm^2 (SATA) for 1 MHz.

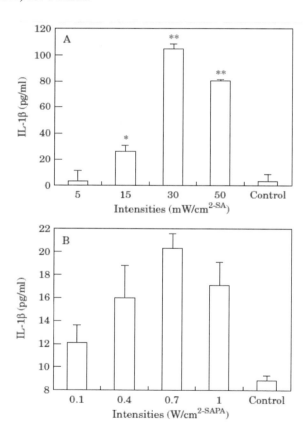

Figure 11.2. Production of interleukin-1β by ultrasound-exposed (a) monocytes, using 45 kHz; and (b) osteoblasts, using 1 MHz (Reprinted from Cytokines, vol. 11, n. 6, Peter Reher, Nghiem Doan, Brian Bradnock, Sajeda Meghji, Malcolm Harris, Effect of ultrasound on the production of IL-8, basic FGF and VEGF, p. 418, Copyright (1999) with permission from Elsevier).

In the same year, Kokubu et al. (1999), based on the hypothesis that LIPUS would have an effect in fracture healing by stimulating the production of the inflammation mediator prostaglandin (PGE_2) from osteoblasts via COX-2 (cyclooxygenase, an enzyme involved in PGE_2 metabolism), aimed at investigating the effect of ultrasound on the level of PGE_2 and COX-2 in mouse osteoblasts. Figure 11.3 depicts the increasing of PGE_2 production by cultured osteoblasts with ultrasound exposure. The authors observed an up-regulation of the expression of COX-2 mRNA (messenger RNA) during the ultrasound stimulation, and the PGE_2 production was suppressed by a selective inhibitor of COX-2 (Figure 11.4), suggesting that the PGE_2 production depends on the induction of COX-2 mRNA expression by ultrasound.

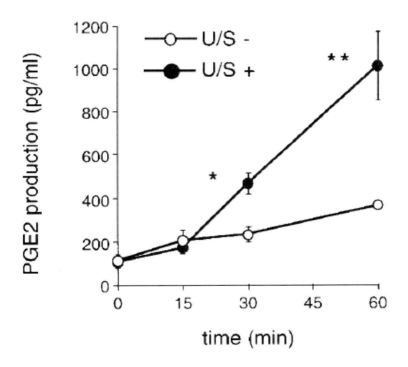

Figure 11.3. Variation in PGE_2 synthesis by cultured osteoblasts cells (with and without ultrasound exposure) in different time points (15, 30 and 60 minutes) (* $p < 0.05$, ** $p < 0.01$) (Reprinted from Biochemical and Biophysical Research Communications, vol. 256, n. 2, Takeshi Kokubu, Nobuzo Matsui, Hiroyuki Fujioka, Masaya Tsunoda, Kosaku Mizuno, Low Intensity Pulsed Ultrasound Exposure Increases Prostaglandin E2 Production via the Induction of Cyclooxygenase-2 mRNA in Mouse Osteoblasts, p. 286, Copyright (1999) with permission from Academic Press).

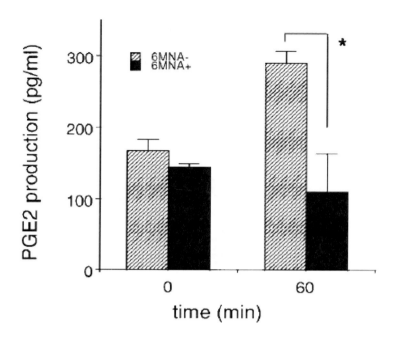

Figure 11.4. The PGE$_2$ production by ultrasound-exposed osteoblasts. 6MNA- and 6MNA+ indicate, respectively, without and with COX-2 inhibitor (* $p < 0.01$) (Reprinted from Biochemical and Biophysical Research Communications, vol. 256, n. 2, Takeshi Kokubu, Nobuzo Matsui, Hiroyuki Fujioka, Masaya Tsunoda, Kosaku Mizuno, Low Intensity Pulsed Ultrasound Exposure Increases Prostaglandin E2 Production via the Induction of Cyclooxygenase-2 mRNA in Mouse Osteoblasts, p. 286, Copyright (1999) with permission from Academic Press).

It is known that the proliferation and differentiation of osteoblasts and chondrocytes are influenced by a calcium-regulating hormone, 1,25-dihydroxyvitamin D$_3$ [1,25-(OH)$_2$D$_3$] (Norman et al., 1982). This evidence led Ito et al. (2000) to examine the effect of LIPUS and 1,25-(OH)$_2$D$_3$ on growth factor secretion in an *in vitro* culture of human osteoblasts and endothelial cells. Ultrasound parameters were: frequency of 1.5 MHz, 200 ms burst sine wave with repeating pulsation at 1.0 kHz, at 30 mW/cm^2 SATA, applied for 20 minutes/day for four consecutive days. Ultrasound and 1,25-(OH)$_2$D$_3$ (including a combination of both) increased the secretion of platelet-derived growth factor (PDGF-AB) (Figure 11.5), showing that ultrasound may accelerate fracture healing by stimulating growth factor secretion from cells in cooperation with 1,25-(OH)$_2$D$_3$.

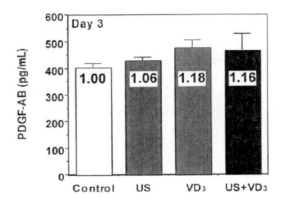

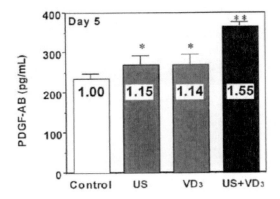

Figure 11.5. Secretion of PDGF-AB in co-cultures of osteoblasts and endothelial cells at day 3 and 5. The numbers inside the columns represent the relative changes compared to the control group. Results for ultrasound (US), 1,25-$(OH)_2D_3$ (VD3) and a combination of both treatments (US+VD$_3$) (* $p < 0.05$; ** $p < 0.01$ compared with control group) (Reprinted from Ultrasound in Medicine & Biology, vol. 26, n. 1, Masaya Ito, Yoshiaki Azuma, Tomohiro Ohita, Keiji Komoriya, Effects of ultrasound and 1,25-dihydroxyvitamin D3 on growth factor secretion in co-cultures of osteoblasts and endothelial cells, p.165, Copyright (2000) with permission from Elsevier).

Naruse et al. (2000) aimed at comparing the anabolic responses in mouse bone marrow stromal cells from ultrasound stimulation. After 20 minutes of ultrasound exposure (1.5 MHz frequency in a pulsed-wave mode, repetition frequency of 1 kHz, at 30 mW/cm^2), a transient expression of an immediate-early gene, c-fos, was observed, presenting the highest value at 40 minutes which subsided by 4 hours. An elevated transient expression of cox-2 message was also obtained. Elevated mRNA levels were observed in many bone proteins (IGF-I, osteocalcin and bone sialoprotein). Figure 11.6 shows mRNA levels of c-fos, growth factors, and bone matrix proteins after a 20 minute ultrasound exposure of bone stromal cells by means of a polimerase chain reaction (PCR) analysis. A similar study was developed by Warden et al. (2001), in which they found a stimulation of the expression of genes c-fos and cox-2, and elevated levels of mRNA for bone matrix proteins alkaline phosphatase (ALP) and osteocalcin.

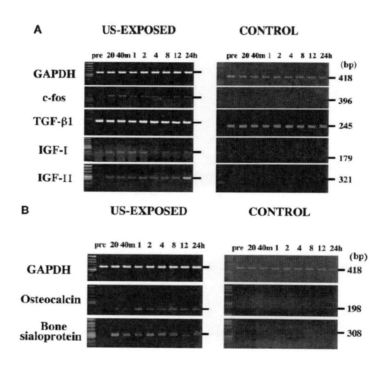

Figure 11.6. Levels of messenger RNA of c-fos, growth factors, and bone matrix proteins for a 20 minutes ultrasound exposure of bone stromal cells (US-exposed) and for a control group. GAPDH (glyceraldehyde 3-phosphate dehydrogenase, an enzyme that catalyzes the sixth step of glycolysis) was used in this study as an internal standard (Reprinted from Biochemical and Biophysical Research Communications, vol. 268, n. 1, Kouji Naruse, Yuko Mikuni-Takagaki, Yoshiaki Azuma, Masaya Ito, Tomohiro Oota, Koh-Zoh Kameyama, Moritoshi Itoman, Anabolic response of mouse bone-marrow-derived stromal cell clone ST2 cells to low-intensity pulsed ultrasound, p. 218, Copyright (2000) with permission from Academic Press).

A study examined the influence of LIPUS on endochondral ossification, using fetal mouse metatarsal rudiments (Nolte et al., 2001). The same ultrasound parameters from the work of Naruse et al. (2000) were used. The ultrasound treatment for 20 minutes/day stimulated the calcification of the diaphysis, and increased the bony collar and the area of calcified hypertrophic cartilage. According to the authors, this effect may be due to an increased activity or an increased number of osteoblasts.

Reher et al. (2002) tried to prove the effect of LIPUS on nitric oxide (NO) induction and prostaglandin E_2 (PGE_2) production in human mandibular osteoblasts *in vitro*, with the same ultrasound parameters from a previous study (Reher et al., 1999). It was observed that ultrasound significantly increased NO and PGE_2 production. With a frequency of 45 kHz, significant stimulation was obtained at 5, 30, and 50 mW/cm^2 SATA. At 1 MHz, the increase was only significant at 0.1 W/cm^2. Figures 11.7 and 11.8 depict the variation in NO and PGE_2 production induced by therapeutic ultrasound.

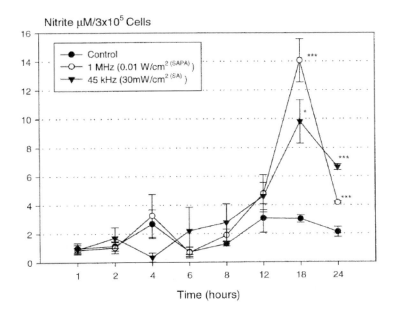

Figure 11.7. Variation in NO production for control and ultrasound at 1 MHz and 45 kHz. The significance levels compared with controls (* $p < 0.05$; ** $p < 0.01$; *** $p < 0.001$) (Reprinted from Bone, vol. 31, n. 1, P. Reher, M. Harris, M. Whiteman, H. K. Hai, S. Meghji, Ultrasound Stimulates Nitric Oxide and Prostaglandin E_2 Production by Human Osteoblasts, p. 238, Copyright (2002) with permission from Elsevier).

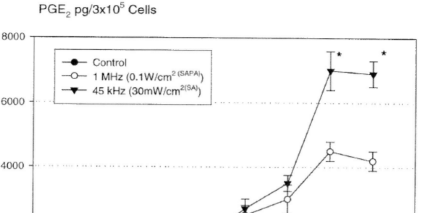

Figure 11.8. Variation in prostaglandin production for control and ultrasound at 1 MHz and 45 kHz. The significance levels compared with controls (* $p < 0.001$) (Reprinted from Bone, vol. 31, n. 1, P. Reher, M. Harris, M. Whiteman, H. K. Hai, S. Meghji, Ultrasound Stimulates Nitric Oxide and Prostaglandin E_2 Production by Human Osteoblasts, p. 239, Copyright (2002) with permission from Elsevier).

Five different ultrasound SATP (spatial-average temporal-peak) intensities (150, 300, 600, 1200 and 2400 mW/cm^2) in far-field exposures, at 1 MHz, were evaluated by Li et al. (2002), to determine their effects on osteoblasts for 15 minutes. Table 11.1 shows the change in osteoblasts cell population after 24 hours of ultrasound stimulation at different intensities. The dose of 600 mW/cm^2 led to a significant difference in cell population ($p < 0.05$) between placebo and treated group. The PGE_2 concentration was increased to approximately 50% (600 mW/cm^2) and 28% (1200 mW/cm^2) from that in the placebo group after 15 minutes of ultrasound stimulation, and the difference between treated and placebo groups presented an ascending tendency from 150 to 600 mW/cm^2 and descending from 600 to 2400 mW/cm^2 (Figure 11.9).

Table 11.1. Change in osteoblasts cell population after 24 hours of ultrasound stimulation at different acoustic intensities (Reprinted from Ultrasound in Medicine & Biology, vol. 28, n. 5, Jimmy Li, Walter Chang, James Lin, Jui-Sheng Sun, Optimum intensities of ultrasound for PGE2 secretion and growth of osteoblasts. Ultrasound Stimulates Nitric Oxide and Prostaglandin E$_2$ Production by Human Osteoblasts, p. 687, Copyright (2002) with permission from Elsevier)

Intensity, mW/cm^2 (I_{SATP})	Sham mean (SD)*	Stimulation mean (SD)*
150	162.93 (11.41)	159.64 (17.88)
300	188.24 (9.80)	193.70 (19.06)
600	186.82 (7.28)	203.37 (8.14)†
1200	201.3 (12.26)	213.59 (13.33)
2400	213.62 (28.87)	211.04 (32.02)

*Sham = osteoblasts were sham treated; stimulation = osteoblasts were treated with ultrasound.
† $p < 0.05$.

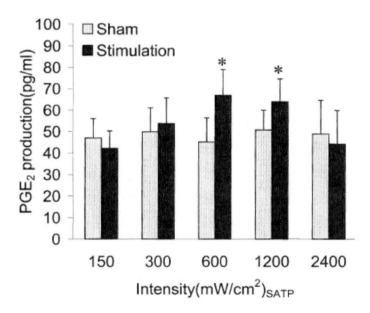

Figure 11.9. Effect of ultrasound of varying intensities on PGE$_2$ synthesis in osteoblasts (Reprinted from Ultrasound in Medicine & Biology, vol. 28, n. 5, Jimmy Li, Walter Chang, James Lin, Jui-Sheng Sun, Optimum intensities of ultrasound for PGE2 secretion and growth of osteoblasts. Ultrasound Stimulates Nitric Oxide and Prostaglandin E$_2$ Production by Human Osteoblasts, p. 687, Copyright (2002) with permission from Elsevier).

Li et al. (2003) verified the effects of ultrasound stimulation on osteoblast growth and cytokine release. They found that the osteoblasts number increased significantly using LIPUS (1 MHz, intensity of 600 mW/cm^2 SATP), 15 minutes/day after only 1-day exposure. The treated cells also presented an increase in TGF-β1 secretion and decrease in concentration of IL-6 and TNF-α. Figures 11.10 and 11.11 show the TNF-α and TGF-β1 concentrations, respectively, for each exposure day. TGF-β1 may have stimulatory effects on osteoblasts, while TNF-α may activate osteoblasts to secrete IL-6 and suppress type-I collagen synthesis (Wrana et al., 1988; Koupa et al., 1999).

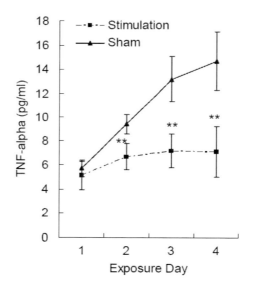

Figure 11.10. TNF-alpha concentrations for each LIPUS exposure day (** = p < 0.01) (Reprinted from Biomaterials, vol. 24, n. 13, J. K. Li, W. H. Chang, J. C. Lin, R. C. Ruaan, H. C. Liu, J. S. Sun, Cytokine release from osteoblasts in response to ultrasound stimulation, p. 2382, Copyright (2003) with permission from Pergamon).

Sant'Anna et al. (2005) developed a study to determine how LIPUS (and a combination with bone morphogenetic proteins - BMP-2) alters gene expression in rat bone marrow stromal cells. An ultrasound operating frequency of 1.5 MHz, and intensity of 30 mW/cm^2 SATA, or sham exposure during 20 minutes was used. A real time PCR was applied to determine gene expression of several genes involved in osteogenesis. Some genes (Cbfa-1/Runx2, IGFreceptor, Alk-3, alkaline phosphatase) presented an increased expression compared to sham controls, and the combination LIPUS/BMP-2 did not lead to a significant synergy.

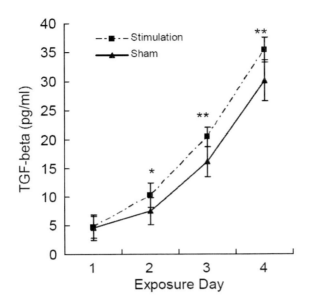

Figure 11.11. TNF-beta concentrations for each LIPUS exposure day (** = p < 0.01) (Reprinted from Biomaterials, vol. 24, n. 13, J. K. Li, W. H. Chang, J. C. Lin, R. C. Ruaan, H. C. Liu, J. S. Sun, Cytokine release from osteoblasts in response to ultrasound stimulation, p. 2383, Copyright (2003) with permission from Pergamon).

An interesting hypothesis was proposed by Hayton et al. (2005). Adenosine 5'-triphosphate (ATP) may be an extracellular signaling molecule in bone tissue; therefore they hypothesized that LIPUS may increase ATP release from osteoblasts, then enhancing fracture healing. Human osteoblasts received ultrasound stimulation, and ATP concentration in the cell culture medium was determined. LIPUS led to increased concentrations of ATP (Figure 11.12). Other results were an increased receptor activator of nuclear factor-kappa B ligand (RANKL), a decreased osteoprotegerin expression and an increased cell proliferation (Figure 11.13).

The so called Wnt/β-catenin signaling pathway is one of the central pathways regulating bone maintenance (Westendorf et al., 2004). Olkku et al. (2010) aimed at characterizing the effects of LIPUS on the activity of Wnt signaling in human osteoblast-like cells. The Wnt signaling pathway was found to be activated following a 10-minutes ultrasound exposure (frequency of 1.035 MHz and intensity of 407 mW/cm^2), showing temperature dependence at elevated temperatures. Cell viability was not affected by neither ultrasound nor heat exposures.

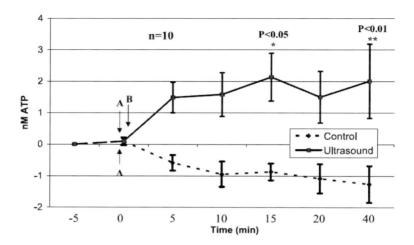

Figure 11.12. ATP release from osteoblasts after ultrasound stimulation (Reprinted from Ultrasound in Medicine & Biology, vol. 31, n. 8, Michael Hayton, Jane Dillon, Danielle Glynn, Judith Curran, James Gallagher, Katherine Buckley, Involvement of adenosine 5'-triphosphate in ultrasound-induced fracture repair, p. 1134, Copyright (2005) with permission from Elsevier).

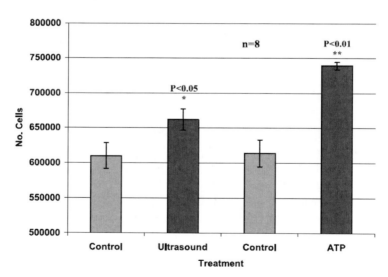

Figure 11.13. The effects of ultrasound and ATP on osteoblast proliferation (number of cells) (Reprinted from Ultrasound in Medicine & Biology, vol. 31, n. 8, Michael Hayton, Jane Dillon, Danielle Glynn, Judith Curran, James Gallagher, Katherine Buckley, Involvement of adenosine 5'-triphosphate in ultrasound-induced fracture repair, p. 1136, Copyright (2005) with permission from Elsevier).

Angle et al. (2011) investigated the effect of LIPUS with intensities lower than 30 mW/cm^2 in provoking phenotypic responses in bone cells. Marrow stromal cells from rats were cultured and insonified with intensities of 2, 15, 30 mW/cm^2 at early, middle and late stages of osteogenic differentiation (cell activation, differentiation into osteogenic cells and biological mineralization, respectively). A rapid increase in the signal for phosphorylated forms of MAPK (mitogen-activated protein kinase) was found with LIPUS intensities of 2, 15 and 30 mW/cm^2, indicating increased phosphorylation compared with the placebo treatment group. Alkaline phosphatase activity, which is an early indicator of osteoblast differentiation, increased by up to 209%, compared to the placebo. The highest increase in mineralization was obtained (225%) in cells treated with 2 mW/cm^2. Increasing intensities dropped the level of mineralization up to 120%. In the same volume of the journal, the research group (Sena et al., 2011) tried to determine: (1) the effect of LIPUS on gap junctional cell-to-cell intercellular communication (important for the function of stromal cells); and (2) whether the ability of bone cells to communicate by gap junctions would affect their response to LIPUS. Rat bone marrow stromal cells (BMSC) were used. A single 20-minutes LIPUS intervention increased the intracellular dye transfer between BMSCs. An addition of gap junction inhibitor, 18β, blocks the transfer of calcein dye, and the presence of 18β diminished the significant increase in ALP activity level by LIPUS stimulation (Figure 11.14).

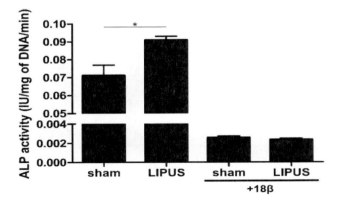

Figure 11.14. ALP activity for sham and LIPUS treatment, and with the presence of 18β, a gap junction inhibitor (Reprinted from Ultrasonics, vol. 51, n. 5, Kotaro Sena, Siddhesh Angle, Arihiko Kanaji, Chetan Aher, David Karwo, Dale Sumner, Amarjit Virdi, Low-intensity pulsed ultrasound (LIPUS) and cell-to-cell communication in bone marrow stromal cells, p. 642, Copyright (2011) with permission from Elsevier).

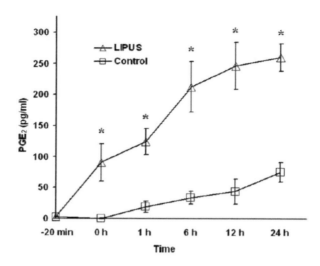

Figure 11.15. PGE$_2$ production induced by a 20-minutes LIPUS in MLO-Y4 cells (* $p < 0.05$) (Reprinted from Biochemical and Biophysical Research Communications, vol. 418, n. 2, Lei Li, Zheng Yang, Hai Zhang, Wenchuan Chen, Mengshi Chen, Zhimin Zhu, Low-intensity pulsed ultrasound regulates proliferation and differentiation of osteoblasts through osteocytes, p. 298, Copyright (2012) with permission from Elsevier).

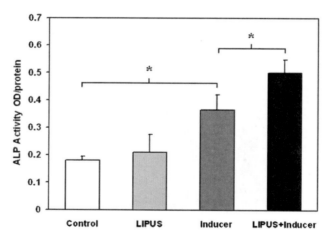

Figure 11.16. ALP activity of MC3T3-E1 cells for each treatment: control, LIPUS, inducers of osteoblast differentiation (ascorbic acid and β-glycerophosphate) and the association of LIPUS + inducer (* $p < 0.05$) (Reprinted from Biochemical and Biophysical Research Communications, vol. 418, n. 2, Lei Li, Zheng Yang, Hai Zhang, Wenchuan Chen, Mengshi Chen, Zhimin Zhu, Low-intensity pulsed ultrasound regulates proliferation and differentiation of osteoblasts through osteocytes, p. 298, Copyright (2012) with permission from Elsevier).

More recently, Li et al. (2012) verified the effect of LIPUS in osteocytic MLO-Y4 cells on proliferation and differentiation of osteoblastic MC3T3-E1 cells. They particularly measured PGE$_2$ and NO secretion from LIPUS-stimulated osteocytes. It was found that LIPUS enhanced secretion of both PGE$_2$ (Figure 11.15) and NO with a 20-minutes exposure from MLO-Y4 cells. Moreover, LIPUS up-regulated ALP activity, and the association of ascorbic acid and β-glycerophosphate significantly increased ALP activity compared to control group (Figure 11.16).

11.3. Animal Models

After the first papers in 1983, proposing LIPUS in animal fracture models as a therapeutic tool (Duarte, 1983; Dyson and Brookes, 1983), Pilla et al. (1990) showed that a daily 20-minute ultrasound stimulation could affect the rate of fibula osteotomy healing in 139 New Zealand rabbits. The contralateral limb was used as a control. Ultrasound parameters were 200-microseconds bursts of 1.5-MHz sine waves, with a repetition frequency at 1.0 kHz, and an intensity of 30 mW/cm^2 SATA. From postoperative day 14 to 23, increases in maximum strength ranged from 40 to 85% ($p \leq 0.01$), and from days 17 to 28, all treated fractures were as strong as intact bones ($p \leq 0.005$). Tsai et al. (1992) tested various acoustic intensities (0.5 and 1.0 W/cm^2 SATA) and treatment durations (5, 15 and 25 minutes/day) also in rabbits, for 4 weeks, using a frequency of 1.5 MHz. The authors showed that a LIPUS at 0.5 W/cm^2 for 15 minutes/day could be used in future studies, and an intensity of 1.0 W/cm^2 was deleterious to the treated fractures.

Wang et al. (1994) worked on bilateral closed femoral shaft fractures in 22 Long-Evans rats. The contralateral limbs served as a control. Ultrasound parameters were a 200 μs burst of 1.5 or 0.5 MHz sine waves, repetition frequency of 1.0 kHz, and intensity of 30 mW/cm^2 SATA. The fractured limb received a daily LIPUS treatment for 15 minutes/day. Radiography, histology and mechanical testing were used to evaluate fracture healing process on postoperative day 21. Both frequencies led to greater values of average maximum torque compared with control limbs ($p < 0.05$), and the 1.5-MHz ultrasound stimulation was able to significantly increase the stiffness of treated fractures ($p < 0.02$).

Two years later, Yang et al. (1996) assessed LIPUS effects on parameters of bone repair after a femur diaphyseal fracture model in 79 Long-Evans rats. The applied ultrasound parameters were the same from Wang et al. (1994), except for the frequency (only 0.5 MHz) and the intensities (50 or 100 mW/cm^2 SATA). Mechanical parameters were significantly greater in treated than in control limbs. Moreover, they observed a shift in the expression of genes associated with cartilage formation in the treated fractures at 50 mW/cm^2, an increase in aggrecan gene expression on day 7 after fracture, and a decrease in the same expression on day 21. Then they suggested that ultrasound could stimulate earlier synthesis of extracellular matrix proteins in cartilage, consequently increasing the mechanical properties of callus tissue.

Takikawa et al. (2001) investigated the effect of LIPUS on nonunion fracture healing in rat tibias. After daily exposures of a 1.5-MHz wave for 20 minutes, and intensity of 30 mW/cm^2 SATA, rats were killed and assessed with radiographs, microfocus X-ray computed tomograms and histologic examination. Results showed that 50% of nonunions were healed on radiologic assessment, after 6 weeks. All control tibias (not treated with ultrasound) remained in a state of nonunion.

Gebauer et al. (2002) evaluated the effect of LIPUS in the enhancement of fracture healing in a diabetes mellitus (type I) rat femoral fracture model. Upon sacrifice, cellular proliferation was assessed using immunohistochemical staining at 2, 4, and 7 days post-fracture, and mechanical testing was also performed. The results showed that there was no influence of ultrasound stimulation on cellular proliferation. However, at six weeks post-fracture, mechanical testing showed a greater torque to failure and stiffness in the US-treated group compared to the control group, corroborating previous findings that ultrasound improves mechanical properties of callus during the late phases of healing.

The role of LIPUS in distraction osteogenesis in rabbits was studied by Uglow et al. (2003), specifically the effect of this treatment on bone mineral content (BMC), density and mechanical properties. After surgery, 4 and 6-weeks tibiae were analyzed using quantitative computed tomography and fourpoint mechanical testing. Histologic analysis was made with two tibiae from each group (treatment and control) at 4 weeks. No significant differences ($p > 0.05$) were observed between groups for BMC, volumetric bone mineral density and cross-sectional area. There was also no significant difference for peak load and modulus of elasticity. Nevertheless, histologic observations showed that the trabecular number decreased, and the trabecular thickness increased in the ultrasound-treated group. The number of osteoclasts was lower in the treated group. Since distraction osteogenesis follows mainly an intramembranous ossification process. These findings indicated that the modulation by ultrasound can occur by accelerating endochondral ossification (via chondrocytes activity).

Hantes et al. (2004) aimed at studying the effect of transosseous application of LIPUS in a midshaft osteotomy of sheep tibiae inserted into the bone, 1.0 cm proximal to the osteotomy site. The 1-Mhz ultrasonic stimulation was made through a free end of a thin stainless-steel pin, with a PZT-4D transducer (average intensity of 30 mW/cm^2 SATA) for 20 minutes daily. Animals were killed and evaluated with mechanical testing and quantitative computed tomography. A significant acceleration of fracture healing in the treated group on radiographic assessment (p = 0.03) was observed. After 75 days, the mean cortical bone mineral density and the ultimate strength were higher in the treated group (p = 0.01).

The effect of different durations of LIPUS treatment were compared during distraction osteogenesis by Chan et al. (2006). New Zealand white rabbit tibiae were osteotomized and lengthened for 1 week. The LIPUS treatment durations were 20 and 40 minutes. Using plain X-rays, quantitative computed tomography and histologic analysis, an increase in bone mineral content and volume, dependent on the ultrasound dose was observed. Corroborating Uglow et al. (2003), LIPUS seemed to enhance endochondral formation.

Li et al. (2007) verified the effect of LIPUS associated with nonsteroidal anti-inflammatory drugs (NSAIDs) in stress fractures induced in ulnae of adult rats. All animals were treated with active-LIPUS in one limb, and inactive-LIPUS in another, after some hours following drug administration. They did not find any interaction between LIPUS and NSAID. LIPUS alone accelerated fracture healing, but the administration of NSAID delayed this process.

An interesting paper published by Perry et al. (2009) studied the effect of ultrasound stimulation on female Wistar rat bone at a physiological level. Three experimental groups were set: (1) application of a cyclic load in the *in vivo* left ulna, in different days; (2) application of a transcutaneous LIPUS to the left ulnae for the same duration as the period of loading; (3) association of loading and ultrasound stimulation. Right ulnae were not loaded serving as a control. For bone assessment, two variables were measured: the proportion of medial periosteal bone surface with double label (dLS/BS%) and the calculation of mineral apposition rate (MAR) from the inter-label distance. The authors have found a significant periosteal response for all three treatments. The association mechanical loading/LIPUS was not significantly different from LIPUS alone.

Shakouri et al. (2010) developed a study with 30 rabbits with mid-tibia open osteotomies, to evaluate the effect of LIPUS on the mineral density and strength of callus. A 1.5-MHz equipment (intensity of 30 mW/cm² SATA) was used in the treated group. They assessed callus development and mineral density with a multidetector computed tomography, and the mechanical properties with three-point bending tests. After 8 weeks of intervention, the treated group presented a higher callus mineral density ($p = 0.001$) in relation to control animals. There was no significant difference between groups concerning mechanical properties.

Although all the evidence supported the use of LIPUS in fracture healing, McClure et al. (2010) performed a randomized, blinded, controlled trial with eight horses. The fracture model was an osteotomy of the right and left fourth metacarpal bone. Daily 40-minutes sessions of LIPUS were done. One fractured bone was used as a control and did not receive ultrasound stimulation. Radiographs were used every week, and after 84 days the bones were collected for an analysis with tomography and histology. The authors found no significant differences between the treated and the control group.

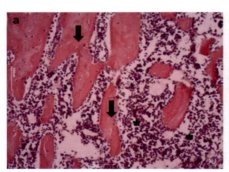 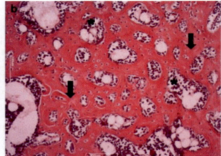

Figure 11.17. Histological analysis after 25 days of surgery from (a) control group and (b) treated group. The asterisks show granulation tissue and the arrows indicate bone tissue. Intense remodeling trabeculae are seen for the treated group (Reprinted from Ultrasound in Medicine & Biology, vol. 36, n. 12, Elaine Fávaro-Pípi, Paulo Bossini, Poliani de Oliveira, Juliana Ribeiro, Carla Tim, Nivaldo Parizotto, José Marcos Alves, Daniel Ribeiro, Heloísa de Araújo, Ana Cláudia Renno, Low-intensity pulsed ultrasound produced an increase of osteogenic genes expression during the process of bone healing in rats, p. 2061, Copyright (2010) with permission from Elsevier).

Fávaro-Pípi et al. (2010) assessed the effect of LIPUS on bone healing in rat tibiae ($n = 60$) using histological analysis and quantitative real-time polymerase chain reaction (qPCR). The animals were divided in two groups: treated and control. Intense new bone formation along with an increased vascularization and osteogenic activity were observed. Figure 11.17 shows the histological analysis after 25 days of surgery from the control and the treated group. It is possible to observe intense remodeling trabeculae for the treated group. After 7 days of postsurgery, an upregulation of genes was also identified (bone morphogenetic protein, osteocalcin and Runx2). Alkaline phosphatase, BMP4 and Runx2 expressions were significantly increased (p < 0.05).

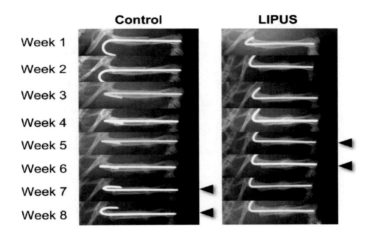

Figure 11.18. Radiographs showing an earlier bone bridging in the LIPUS group (weeks 5 and 6) compared with the control group (weeks 7 and 8) (Reprinted from Ultrasound in Medicine & Biology, vol. 37, n. 2, Wing-Hoi Cheung, Simon Kwoon-Ho Chow, Ming-Hui Sun, Ling Qin, Kwok-Sui Leung, Low-intensity pulsed ultrasoundaccelerated callus formation, angiogenesis and callus remodeling in osteoporotic fracture healing, p. 233, copyright (2011) with permission from Elsevier).

A group from China has recently done a remarkable study in this field. First of all, Cheung et al. (2011) used ovariectomy-induced osteoporotic fractures in rats to evaluate the therapeutic effects of LIPUS. The animals were assessed by gene expression quantification, radiographic and histological analysis. Radiographs showed that LIPUS accelerated fracture healing compared with the control group (Figure 11.18). A greater callus area and increased callus size were also observed with significant difference. Histological analysis showed a stronger signal of cartilaginous tissue and a larger area of callus in the LIPUS group (at week 2), an increase in the calcified tissue and endochondral ossification (at week 4) and a smaller area of callus and cartilage compared with the control animals (at week 8), as seen in Figure 11.19. In the same year and journal, they hypothesized that LIPUS effects could be optimized by adjusting the incidence critical angle to the surface of bone, using a rat femoral fracture model (n = 100). The authors found that the callus mineralization, bridging and biomechanical properties were significantly enhanced using a critical angle of 35° after 8 weeks post-surgery (Table 11.2 and Figure 11.20) (Chung et al., 2011).

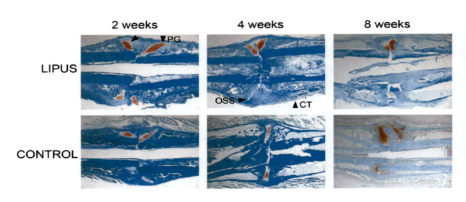

Figure 11.19. Histological qualitative analysis showing the fracture gap for LIPUS and control groups. A higher content in cartilage (PG = proteoglycan signal) was seen at week 2. Calcified tissue increased (arrows) at week 4 (OSS = site of endochondral ossification; CT = calcified tissue). At week 8, LIPUS produced a decrease in the amounts of cartilage (Reprinted from Ultrasound in Medicine & Biology, vol. 37, n. 2, Wing-Hoi Cheung, Simon Kwoon-Ho Chow, Ming-Hui Sun, Ling Qin, Kwok-Sui Leung, Low-intensity pulsed ultrasoundaccelerated callus formation, angiogenesis and callus remodeling in osteoporotic fracture healing, p. 236, copyright (2011) with permission from Elsevier).

Table 11.2. Percentage of complete mineralized callus bridging of ultrasound-treated animals at different incident angles (0°, 35°, 22° and 48°) assessed by radiographs. In 35° group, the callus bridged at 8 weeks in 90,90% of the samples (Reprinted from Ultrasound in Medicine & Biology, vol. 37, n. 7, Shu Chung, Neill Pounder, Francisco de Ana, Ling Qin, Kwok Leung, Wing Cheung, Fracture healing enhancement with low intensity pulsed ultrasound at a critical application angle, p. 1126, Copyright (2011) with permission from Elsevier)

	Weeks after treatment			
Group	5	6	7	8
Control	0%	9.10%	27.30%	36.30%
0°	0%	9.10%	27.30%	45.50%
35°	18.20%	54.50%	81.80%	90.90%
22°	36.40%	63.60%	63.60%	63.60%
48°	0%	27.30%	54.50%	72.70%

Therapeutic Ultrasound in Fractures: State of the Art 237

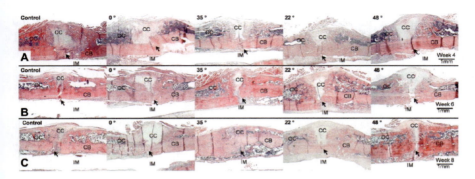

Figure 11.20. Histomorphologic analysis of the callus from the control group with placebo treatment and groups treated with LIPUS at different incident angles at weeks 4, 6 and 8 (A, B and C, respectively). It is possible to observe an earlier remodeling of woven bone, as well as a complete bridging of newly woven bone in the 35° group. CC = cartilaginous callus; OC = osseous callus; CB = cortical bone; IM = intramedullary canal. The arrows indicate the fracture site (Reprinted from Ultrasound in Medicine & Biology, vol. 37, n. 7, Shu Chung, Neill Pounder, Francisco de Ana, Ling Qin, Kwok Leung, Wing Cheung, Fracture healing enhancement with low intensity pulsed ultrasound at a critical application angle, p. 1130, Copyright (2011) with permission from Elsevier).

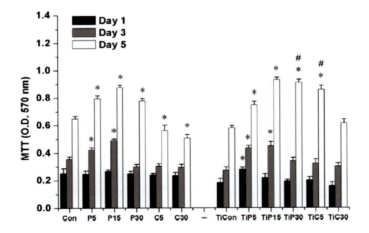

Figure 11.21. Cell viability by inhibition of 3-(4,5-Dimethylthiazol-2-yl)-2,5-diphenyltetrazolium bromide (MTT) reduction for all the experimental groups (Con = control; P5 = pulse 0.05 W/cm²; P15 = pulse 0.15 W/cm²; P30 = pulse 0.30 W/cm²; C5 = continuous 0.05 W/cm²; C30 = continuous 0.30 W/cm²; Ti indicates the viability of the MG63 cells attached to the Cp-Ti plates) (Reprinted from Ultrasound in Medicine & Biology, vol. 37, n. 3, Shih-Kuang Hsu, Wen-Tao Huang, Bai-Shuan Liu, Shih-Miao Li, Hsien-Te Chen, Chen-Jung Chang, Effects of near-field ultrasound stimulation on new bone formation and osseointegration of dental titanium implants in vitro and in vivo, p. 409, Copyright (2011) with permission from Elsevier).

Hsu et al. (2011) performed an *in vitro* and *in vivo* study (New Zealand rabbits) to analyze the effect of a near-field ultrasound stimulation system (1 MHz, continuous and pulse, intensities from 0.05 to 0.30 W/cm² SATA, 10 minutes daily) to enhance the osseointegration of the dental titanium implant into the adjacent bone. A commercially pure titanium (Cp-Ti) plate was placed in a cultured rat neonatal calvarial defect (*in vitro* model) whereas CP-Ti implants were inserted into the metaphysis of rabbit tibia (*in vivo* model). Assessment was made by using histomorphometric and image analysis, including color Doppler ultrasonography to identify blood flow supplies. LIPUS enhanced cell migration and new bone regeneration. Moreover, an acceleration in bone formation was observed(Figure 11.21 shows cell viability in response to LIPUS), as well as a greater proliferation of blood flow and mature type I collagen fibers.

In a more recent paper comparing different intensities of LIPUS in rats, Fung et al. (2012) verified that a LIPUS at 30 mW/cm² presented a significantly higher low-density bone volume fraction and woven bone percentage than that of the control group and LIPUS at 150 mW/cm². The failure torque of LIPUS at 30 mW/cm² was significantly higher than the control group and LIPUS-150 after 6 weeks post-surgery.

11.4. Clinical Studies

Several systematic reviews and meta-analysis have been published in the last years presenting the evidence that support the use of LIPUS in fracture healing (Siska et al., 2008; Gleizal et al., 2011; Watanabe et al., 2010; Albornoz et al., 2011). More recently, a meta-analysis performed by Tajali et al. (2012) focused on clinical trials, using as inclusion criteria: human clinical trials, all types of bones/fractures and outcome measurements, the use of LIPUS, and papers written in English. Twenty-three studies were selected and divided into three groups: fresh fractures, delayed or nonunions, and distraction osteogenesis. The criterion for the meta-analysis was the time of the third cortical bridging, which is the increase in density or size of initial periosteal reaction. The authors concluded that LIPUS stimulates the radiographic bone healing in fresh fractures. Weak evidence could be observed for delayed unions and nonunions and distraction osteogenesis. Nevertheless, it is important to say here that some papers have also been published showing no significant differences between treated and non-treated groups.

Some of the studies from the last 10 years will be highlighted here. Important previous research is worth mentioning, for example, from Heckman et al. (1994), Kristiansen et al. (1997), Cook et al. (1997), Mayr et al. (2000), and Nolte et al. (2001), who pointed out the acceleration of fracture healing with LIPUS (although the paper of Emami et al., in 2000, suggesting that LIPUS has not significantly reduced the healing time in fresh tibial fractures treated with a reamed intramedullary nailing).

Leung et al. (2004) conducted a clinical trial to verify the effect of a daily 20-minutes LIPUS on tibial fractures, with thirty patients randomly assigned to two groups: treated and sham. Internal or external fixations were used according to each case. There was significantly better healing in the LIPUS-treated group, and complications were minimal in these patients. One case of delayed union was observed in each group, and two cases of infection in the placebo group.

Tsumaki et al. (2004) aimed at determining if LIPUS would accelerate fracture healing after hemocallotasis (a procedure where the bone - usually in proximal tibia - is cut through half its width and then the two parts are slowly distracted using an external fixator) in elderly patients. The sample consisted of twenty-one subjects with osteoarthritis and similar degrees of knee varus deformity. During four weeks, callus bone mineral density was significantly greater in the ultrasound-treated tibiae than in the control group ($p = 0.02$). In the same year, Rue et al. (2004) conducted a prospective, randomized, double-blind trial to determine the effect of LIPUS on tibial stress fractures in twenty-six midshipmen (an officer cadet or a commissioned officer). They were randomized to treated and placebo groups. Daily interventions were continued until patients were asymptomatic with radiographic signs of healing. However, there was no significant difference between groups for all the parameters considered (for example, delay from symptom onset to diagnosis, missed treatment days, total number of treatments, and time to return to duty). The authors did not use any other specific parameter for monitoring.

In 2005, several studies were published in this domain. Handolin et al. (2005) presented three papers with the same objective: to verify the effect of LIPUS associated with bioabsorbable self-reinforced poly-L-lactide (SR-PLLA) screw fixation on the bone in lateral malleolar fractures. Dual-energy X-ray absorptiometry (DXA) and radiographs were used to evaluate bone mineral density and bone healing, respectively. There was no significant difference between treated and non-treated group. A good biocompatibility between the bioabsorbable SR-PLLA screw and LIPUS was observed. Gold and Wasserman (2005) applied LIPUS on patients after a distraction osteogenesis. The sample was composed of eight patients with large tibial segmental defects. Each tibial defect was stimulated for 20 minutes daily. Two outcome parameters were used: the external fixation time (in months) and the external fixation index (in months per cm). Although they found a reduction of 17.21% in the external fixation index for the treated group, no significant difference was obtained between treated and control groups. El-Mowafi and Mohsen (2005) also used LIPUS in distraction osteogenesis, managing 20 patients with tibial defects ranging from 5 to 8 cm. Radiographs were used to monitor all patients every week, to identify the formation of an external cortex and an intramedullary canal, finally removing the fixator. The mean healing index in group A was 30 days/cm, while in group B it was 48 days/cm ($p < 0.001$). Nevertheless, a study of Schortinghuis et al. (2005) with eight patients who underwent a mandibular vertical distraction showed no significant difference between treated and placebo groups regarding the mean area of mineralised tissue (by microradiographic examination of biopsies) and histological analysis.

Rutten et al. (2007) aimed at determining the effect of LIPUS on tibia nonunions. Seventy-one cases have been included. It was obtained an overall healing rate of 73%, as well as a statistical significant higher healing rate compared to literature ($p < 0.0001$). During a reanalysis of previously published data on LIPUS treatment for postoperative delayed union and nonunion, Jingushi et al. (2007) verified that there was a significant relationship between the union rate and the time when a radiological improvement was first observed after the beginning of LIPUS treatment. Besides, 89.7% of all fractures healed with LIPUS treatment starting within 6 months. Regarding an improvement in radiological findings, the sensitivity and specificity for union were more than 90%.

Lubbert et al. (2008) evaluated LIPUS on clavicle shaft fractures with a randomised double blind, placebo-controlled multi-centre trial. A total of 101 adult patients were enrolled, and divided into two groups: placebo and active LIPUS groups. No differences were obtained in Visual Analogue Pain Scores (VAS), time to subjective clinical fracture healing, resumption of daily activities, and use of pain medication.

The effect of LIPUS on delayed union was again considered by Rutten et al. (2008) with thirteen patients with osteotomized fibula. A randomized prospective double-blind placebo-controlled trial was performed. Histomorphometrical analysis provided information about bone formation, bone resorption and angiogenesis. The authors found a significantly increase in osteoid thickness (47%), mineral apposition rate (27%) and bone volume

(33%) in LIPUS-treated group. No effect in angiogenesis was observed. In a multi-center randomized sham-controlled trial (Schofer et al., 2010) with 51 patients with tibial delayed union, the authors verified that the estimated increase in bone mineral density in the LIPUS group was 34% larger than in the placebo group. Besides, LIPUS led to a significantly smaller residual gap area at the fracture site.

Finally, Dudda et al. (2011) aimed at determining whether the use of LIPUS during callus distraction results in accelerated mineralization of the regenerated bone formation and a shortened treatment time. Safety of treatment with LIPUS was also monitored in 36 patients. Standard radiographs were used to assess bone regeneration by every 3 to 4 weeks, and all patients were scored by two indexes: the distraction consolidation index (the ratio of fixator gestation time in days over the distraction gap size in centimeters, given in days/cm) and the Paley index (ratio of fixator gestation period in months over the distraction gap size in centimeters, given in months/cm). There were no significant differences between groups; however the authors found that the fixator gestation period could be decreased for 43.6 days in the treatment group.

Conclusion

Ultrasound undoubtedly has some effect in fracture healing. Most of the evidence (*in vitro*, animal models and human clinical trials) have shown that acoustic waves seem to stimulate osteoblasts to produce inflammatory mediators like TGF, nitric oxide, prostaglandins etc. The genetic expression in stromal cells can be increased. Histological analysis, coupled with other imaging modalities (simple radiographs, microtomography) and mechanical tests have demonstrated that animals treated with LIPUS recover bone function in a period of time shorter that in the control or the placebo group. Clinical trials have already found successful results in several fractures and complications.

LIPUS (applied to bone fractures) has been a very attractive research subject. First of all, ultrasound seems to cause no harm (at least there is no evidence reporting problems in the case of infection, osteosynthesis, or metallic devices). The use of ultrasound could avoid surgical procedures in many cases. On the other hand, researchers have observed an enhancement in fracture healing in specific clinical situations like fresh fractures and nonunions.

In the future, studies have to focus essentially on the explanation of how ultrasound affects fracture healing phenomenon *in vivo*: does it act only at a cellular level, increasing mesenchymal cells and osteoblasts activity? Is there a significant increase in temperature capable of stimulating cellular metabolism? Would LIPUS have also an effect on the increase of vascularization? Which would be the effects of a metal nailing or screws inside the bone tissue during ultrasound stimulation?

Another point to be discussed: mainly all the studies used a "near-field stimulation", i.e., an unfocused transducer is placed in contact with skin, stimulating the tissues inside the ultrasonic near field (Chapter 4). It is known that the intensity varies along the beam axis inside the near field. So would the stimulation with a focused transducer be more effective than with an unfocused one?

These questions have to be raised and answered in the near future; meanwhile, researchers worldwide are continuing to make these efforts.

References

Albornoz, P. M., Khanna, A., Longo, U. G., Forriol, F., & Maffuli, N. (2011). The evidence of low-intensity pulsed ultrasound for in vitro, animal and human fracture healing. *British Medical Bulletin, 100*, 39-57.

Angle, S. R., Sena, K., Sumner, D. R., & Virdi, A. S. (2011). Osteogenic differentiation of rat bone marrow stromal cells by various intensities of low-intensity pulsed ultrasound. *Ultrasonics, 51*, 281-288.

Chan, C. W., Qin, L., Lee, K. M., Cheung, W. H., Cheng, J. C., Leung, K. S. (2006). Dose-dependent effect of low-intensity pulsed ultrasound on callus formation during rapid distraction osteogenesis. *Journal of Orthopaedical Research, 24*, 2072–2079.

Chapman, I. V., MacNally, N. A., & Tucker, S. (1980). Ultrasound-induced changes in rates of influx and efflux of potassium ions in rat thymocytes in vitro. *Ultrasound in Medicine & Biology, 6*, 47-58.

Cheung, W.-H., Chow, S. K.-H., Sun, M.-H., Qin, L., & Leung, K.-S. (2011). Low-intensity pulsed ultrasoundaccelerated callus formation, angiogenesis and callus remodeling in osteoporotic fracture healing. *Ultrasound in Medicine & Biology, 37*, 231-238.

Chung, S. L., Pounder, N. M., de Ana, F. J., Qin, L., Leung, K. S., & Cheung, W. H. (2011). Fracture healing enhancement with low intensity pulsed ultrasound at a critical application angle. *Ultrasound in Medicine & Biology, 37,* 1120-1133.

Cook, S. D., Ryaby, J. P., McCabe, J., Frey, J. J., Heckman, J. D., & Kristiansen, T. K. (1997). Acceleration of tibia and distal radius fracture healing in patients who smoke. *Clinical Orthopaedics and Related Research, 337,* 198-207.

Corradi, C., & Cozzolino, A. (1953). Ultrasound and bone callus formation during function. *Arch Ortop, 66,* 77-98.

Doan, N., Reher, P., Meghji, S., & Harris, M. (1999). In vitro effects of therapeutic ultrasound on cell proliferation, protein synthesis, and cytokine production by human fibroblasts, osteoblasts, and monocytes. *Journal of Oral and Maxillofacial Surgery, 57,* 409-419.

Duarte, L. R. (1983). The stimulation of bone growth by ultrasound. Archives of Orthopaedic and Traumatic Surgery, 101, 153-159.

Dudda, M., Hauser, J., Muhr, G., & Esenwein, S. A. (2011). Low-intensity pulsed ultrasound as a useful adjuvant during distraction osteogenesis: a prospective, randomized controlled trial. *The Journal of Trauma, 71,* 1376-1380.

Dyson, M., & Brookes, M. (1983). Stimulation of bone repair by ultrasound. *Ultrasound in Medicine & Biology, Suppl. 2,* 61-66.

Emami, A., Petrén-Mallmin, M., & Larsson, S. (1999). No effect of low-intensity ultrasound on healing time of intramedullary fixed tibial fractures. *Journal of Orthopaedic Trauma, 13,* 252-257.

Fávaro-Pípi, E., Bossini, P., Oliveira, P., Ribeiro, J. U., Tim, C., Parizotto, N. A., Alves, J. M., Ribeiro, D. A., Araújo, H. S. S., & Renno, A. C. M. (2010). Low-intensity pulsed ultrasound produced an increase of osteogenic genes expression during the process of bone healing in rats. *Ultrasound in Medicine & Biology, 36,* 2057-2064.

Fung, C.-H., Cheung, W.-H., Pounder, N. M., de Ana, F. J., Harrison, A., & Leung, K.-S. (2012). Effects of different therapeutic ultrasound intensities on fracture healing in rats. *Ultrasound Medicine & Biology, 38,* 745-752.

Gebauer, G. P., Lin, S. S., Beam, H. A., Vieira, P., & Parsons, J. R. (2002). Low-intensity pulsed ultrasound increases the fracture callus strength in diabetic BB Wistar rats but does not affect cellular proliferation. *Journal of Orthopaedic Research, 20,* 587-592.

Gleizal, A., Lavandier, B., Paris, M., & Béra, J.-C. (2011). Intérêt des ultrasons pulsés de faible intensité dans la stimulation de la régénération osseuse. *Revue de Stomatologie et de Chirurgie Maxillofaciale, 112*, 233-239.

Gold, S. M., & Wasserman, R. (2005). Preliminary results of tibial bone transports with pulsed low intensity ultrasound (Exogen). *Journal of Orthopaedic Trauma, 19*, 10-16.

Hadjiargyrou, M., McLeod, K., Ryaby, J. P., & Rubin, C. (1998). Enhancement of fracture healing by low intensity ultrasound. *Clinical Orthopaedics and Related Research, 355S*, S216-S229.

Handolin, L., Kiljunen, V., Arnala, I., Kiuru, M. J., Pajarinen, J., Partio, E. K., & Rokkanen, P. (2005). Effect of ultrasound therapy on bone healing of lateral malleolar fractures of the ankle joint fixed with bioabsorbable screws. *Journal of Orthopaedic Science, 10*, 391-395.

Handolin, L., Kiljunen, V., Arnala, I., Kiuru, M. J., Pajarinen, J., Partio, E. K., & Rokkanen, P. (2005). No long-term effects of ultrasound therapy on bioabsorbable screw-fixed lateral malleolar fracture. *Scandinavian Journal of Surgery, 94*, 239-242.

Handolin, L., Kiljunen, V., Arnala, I., Pajarinen, J., Partio, E. K., & Rokkanen, P. (2005). The effect of low intensity ultrasound and bioabsorbable self-reinforced poly-L-lactide screw fixation on bone in lateral malleolar fractures. *Archives of Orthopaedic Trauma and Surgery, 125*, 317-321.

Hantes, M. E., Mavrodontidis, A. N., Zalavras, C. G., Karantanas, A. H., Karachalios, & Malizos, K. N. (2004). Low intensity transosseous ultrasound accelerates osteotomy healing in a sheep fracture model. *Journal of Bone and Joint Surgery American Volume, 86-A*, 2275–82.

Hayton, M. J., Dillon, J. P., Glynn, D., Curran, J. M., Gallagher, J. A., & Buckley, K. A. (2005). Involvement of adenosine 5'-triphosphate in ultrasound-induced fracture repair. *Ultrasound in Medicine & Biology, 31*, 1131-1138.

Heckman, J. D., Ryaby, J. P., McCabe, J., Frey, J. J., & Kilcoyne, R. F. (1994). Acceleration of tibial fracture-healing by non-invasive, low-intensity pulsed ultrasound. *The Journal of Bone and Joint Surgery - American Volume, 76*, 26-34.

Hsu, S.-K., Huang, W.-T., Liu, B.-S., Li, S.-M., Chen, H.-T., & Chang, C.-J. (2011). Effects of near-field ultrasound stimulation on new bone formation and osseointegration of dental titanium implants in vitro and in vivo. *Ultrasound in Medicine & Biology, 37*, 403-416.

Ito, M., Azuma, Y., Ohta, T., & Komoriya, K. (2000). Effects of ultrasound and 1,25-dihydroxyvitamin D3 on growth factor secretion in co-cultures of osteoblasts and endothelial cells. *Ultrasound in Medicine & Biology, 26*, 161-166.

Jingushi, S., Mizuno, K., Matsushita, T., & Itoman, M. (2007). Low-intensity pulsed ultrasound treatment for postoperative delayed union or nonunion of long bone fractures. *Journal of Orthopaedic Science, 12*, 35-41.

Kokubu, T., Matsui, N., Fujioka, H., Tsunoda, M., & Mizuno, K. (1999). Low Intensity Pulsed Ultrasound Exposure Increases Prostaglandin E2 Production via the Induction of Cyclooxygenase-2 mRNA in Mouse Osteoblasts. *Biochemical and Biophysical Research Communications, 256*, 284–287.

Kouba, D. J., Chung, K. Y., Nishiyama, T., Vindevoghel, L., Kon, A., Klement, J. F., Uitto, J., & Mauviel, A. (1999). Nuclear factor-kappa B mediates TNF-alpha inhibitory effect on alpha 2(I) collagen (COL1A2) gene transcription in human dermal fibroblasts. *Journal of Immunology, 162*, 4226-4234.

Kristiansen, T. K., Ryaby, J. P., McCabe, J., Frey, J. J., & Roe, L. R. (1997). Accelerated healing of distal radial fractures with the use of specific, low-intensity ultrasound. A multicenter, prospective, randomized, double-blind, placebo-controlled study. *The Journal of Bone and Joint Surgery - American Volume, 79*, 961-973.

Leung, K. S., Lee, W. S., Tsui, H. F., Liu, P. P., & Cheung, W. H. (2004). Complex tibial fracture outcomes following treatment with low-intensity pulsed ultrasound. *Ultrasound in Medicine & Biology, 30*, 389-395.

Li, J. G.-R., Chang, W. H.-S., Lin, J. C.-A., & Sun, J.-S. (2002). Optimum intensities of ultrasound for PGE_2 secretion and growth of osteoblasts. *Ultrasound in Medicine & Biology, 28*, 683-690.

Li, J. K., Chang, W. H., Lin, J. C., Ruaan, R. C., Liu, H. C., & Sun, J. S. (2003). Cytokine release from osteoblasts in response to ultrasound stimulation. *Biomaterials, 24*, 2379-2385.

Li, J., Waugh, L. J., Hui, S. L., Burr, D. B., & Warden, S. J. (2007). Low-intensity pulsed ultrasound and nonsteroidal anti-inflammatory drugs have opposing effects during stress fracture repair. *Journal of Orthopaedical Research, 25*, 1559-1567.

Li, L., Yang, Z., Zhang, H., Chen, W., Chen, M., & Zhu, Z. (2012). Low-intensity pulsed ultrasound regulates proliferation and differentiation of osteoblasts through osteocytes. *Biochemical and Biophysical Research Communications, 418*, 296–300.

Lubbert, P. H., van der Rijt, R. H., Hoorntje, L. E., & van der Werken, C. (2008). Low-intensity pulsed ultrasound (LIPUS) in fresh clavicle fractures: a multi-centre double blind randomised controlled trial. *Injury, 39*, 1444-1452.

Maintz, G. (1950). Tierexperimentelle untersuchungen uber dle wirkung der ultraschallwellen auf die knochenregeneration. *Strahlentherapie, 82*, 631-638.

Mayr, E., Frankel, V., & Rüter, A. (2000). Ultrasound - an alternative healing method for nonunions? *Archives of Orthopaedic and Trauma Surgery, 120(1-2)*, 1-8.

McClure, S. R., Miles, K., Vansickle, D., & South, T. (2010). The effect of variable waveform low-intensity pulsed ultrasound in a fourth metacarpal osteotomy gap model in horses. *Ultrasound Medicine & Biology, 36*, 1298-1305.

Naruse, K., Mikuni-Takagaki, Y., Azuma, Y., Ito, M., Oota, T., Kameyama, K.-Z., & Itoman, M. (2000). Anabolic Response of Mouse Bone-Marrow-Derived Stromal Cell Clone ST2 Cells to Low-Intensity Pulsed Ultrasound. *Biochemical and Biophysical Research Communications, 268*, 216–220.

Nolte, P. A., Klein-Nulend, J., Albers, G. H. R., Marti, R. K., Semeins, C. M., Goei, S. W., & Burger, E. H. (2001). Low-intensity ultrasound stimulates endochondral ossification in vitro. *Journal of Orthopaedic Research, 19*, 301-307.

Nolte, P. A., van der Krans, A., Patka, P., Janssen, I. M., Ryaby, J. P., & Albers, G. H. (2001). Low-intensity pulsed ultrasound in the treatment of nonunions. *The Journal of Trauma, 51*, 693-702.

Norman, A. W., Roth, J., & Orci, L. (1982). The vitamin D endocrine system: steroid metabolism, hormone receptors, and biological response (calcium binding proteins). *Endocrine Reviews, 3*, 331-336.

Olkku, A., Leskinen, J. J., Lammi, M. J., Hynynen, K., & Mahonen, A. (2010). Ultrasound-induced activation of Wnt signaling in human MG-63 osteoblastic cells. *Bone, 47*, 320-330.

Parvizi, J., Parpura, V., Kinnick, R. R., Greenleaf, J. F., & Bolander, M. E. (1997). Low intensity ultrasound increases intracellular concentration of calcium in chondrocytes. *Transactions of the Orthopaedic Research Society, 22*, 465.

Perry, M. J., Parry, L. K., Burton, V. J., Gheduzzi, S., Beresford, J. N., Humphrey, V. F., & Skerry, T. M. (2009). Ultrasound mimics the effect of mechanical loading on bone formation in vivo on rat ulnae. *Medical Engineering & Physics, 31*, 42-47.

Pilla, A. A., Mont, M. A., Nasser, P. R., Khan, S. A., Figueiredo, M., Kaufman, J. J., & Siffert, R. S. (1990). Non-invasive low-intensity pulsed ultrasound accelerates bone healing in the rabbit. *Journal of Orthopaedic Trauma, 4*, 246-253.

Reher, P., Elbeshir, E.-N., Harvey, W., Meghji, S., & Harris, M. (1997). The stimulation of bone formation in vitro by therapeutic ultrasound. *Ultrasound in Medicine & Biology, 23*, 1251-1258.

Reher, P., Doan, N., Bradnock, B., Meghji, S., & Harris, M. (1999). Effect of ultrasound on the production of IL-8, basic FGF and VEGF. *Cytokines, 11*, 416-423.

Reher, P., Harris, M., Whiteman, M., Hai, H. K., & Meghji, S. (2002). Ultrasound stimulates nitric oxide and prostaglandin E_2 production by human osteoblasts. *Bone, 31*, 236-241.

Rue, J. P., Armstrong, D. W., Frassica, F. J., Deafenbaugh, M., & Wilckens, J. H. (2004). The effect of pulsed ultrasound in the treatment of tibial stress fractures. *Orthopedics, 27*, 1192-1195.

Rutten, S., Nolte, P. A., Guit, G. L., Bouman, D. E., & Albers, G. H. (2007). Use of low-intensity pulsed ultrasound for posttraumatic nonunions of the tibia: a review of patients treated in the Netherlands. *The Journal of Trauma, 62*, 902-908.

Rutten, S., Nolte, P. A., Korstjens, C. M., van Duin, M. A., & Klein-Nulend, J. (2008). Low-intensity pulsed ultrasound increases bone volume, osteoid thickness and mineral apposition rate in the area of fracture healing in patients with a delayed union of the osteotomized fibula. *Bone, 43*, 348-354.

Ryaby, J. T., Mathew, J., & Duarte-Alves, P. (1992). Low intensity pulsed ultrasound affects adenylate cyclase activity and TGF-β synthesis in osteoblastic cells. *Transactions of the Orthopaedic Research Society, 7*, 590.

Sant'Anna, E. F., Leven, R. M., Virdi, A. S., & Sumner, D. R. (2005). Effect of low intensity pulsed ultrasound and BMP-2 on rat bone marrow stromal cell gene expression. *Journal of Orthopaedic Research, 23*, 646-652.

Schofer, M. D., Block, J. E., Aigner, J., & Schmelz, A. (2010). Improved healing response in delayed unions of the tibia with low-intensity pulsed ultrasound: results of a randomized sham-controlled trial. *BMC Musculoskeletal Disorders, 11*, 229-234.

Schortinghuis, J., Bronckers, A. L., Stegenga, B., Raghoebar, G. M., & de Bont, L. G. (2005). Ultrasound to stimulate early bone formation in a distraction gap: a double blind randomised clinical pilot trial in the edentulous mandible. *Archives of Oral Biology, 50*, 411-420.

Sena, K., Angle, S. R., Kanaji, A., Aher, C., Karwo, D. G., Sumner, D. R., & Virdi, A. S. (2011). Low-intensity pulsed ultrasound (LIPUS) and cell-to-cell communication in bone marrow stromal cells. *Ultrasonics, 51*, 639-644.

Shakouri, K., Eftekharsadat, B., Oskuie, M. R., Soleimanpour, J., Tarzamni, M. K., Salekzamani, Y., Hoshyar, Y., & Nezami, N. (2010). Effect of low-intensity pulsed ultrasound on fracture callus mineral density and flexural strength in rabbit tibial fresh fracture. *Journal of Orthopedical Science, 15*, 240-244.

Siska, P. A., Gruen, G. S., & Pape, H. C. (2008). External adjuncts to enhance fracture healing: what is the role of ultrasound? *Injury, 39*, 1095-1105.

Tajali, S. B., Houghton, P., MacDermid, J. C., & Grewal, R. (2012). Effects of low-intensity pulsed ultrasound therapy on fracture healing: a systematic review and meta-analysis. *American Journal of Physical Medicine & Rehabilitation, 91*, 349-367.

Takikawa, S., Matsui, N., Kokubu, T., Tsunoda, M., Fujioka, H., Mizuno, K., & Azuma, Y. (2001). Low-intensity pulsed ultrasound initiates bone healing in rat nonunion fracture model. *Journal of Ultrasound in Medicine, 20*, 197–205.

Tsai, C. L., Chang, W. H., & Liu, T. K. (1992). Preliminary studies of duration and intensity of ultrasonic treatments on fracture repair. *The Chinese Journal of Physiology, 35*, 21-26.

Tsumaki, N., Kakiuchi, M., Sasaki, J., Ochi, T., & Yoshikawa, H. (2004). Low-intensity pulsed ultrasound accelerates maturation of callus in patients treated with opening-wedge high tibial osteotomy by hemicallotasis. *The Journal of Bone and Joint Surgery - American Volume, 86-A*, 2399-2405.

Uglow, M. G., Peat, R. A., Hile, M. S., Bilston, L. E., Smith, E. J., & Little, D. (2003). Low-intensity ultrasound stimulation in distraction osteogenesis in rabbits. *Clinical Orthopedics and Related Research, 417*, 303–12

Wang, S. J., Lewallen, D. G., Bolander, M. E., Chao, E. Y., Ilstrup, D. M., & Greenleaf, J. F. (1994). Low intensity ultrasound treatment increases strength in a rat femoral fracture model. *Journal of Orthopaedic Research, 12,* 40-47.

Warden, S. J., Favaloro, J. M., Bennell, K. L., McMeeken, J. M., Ng, Kong-Wah, Zajac, J. D., & Wark, J. D. (2001). Low-Intensity Pulsed Ultrasound Stimulates a Bone-Forming Response in UMR-106 Cells. *Biochemical and Biophysical Research Communications, 286,* 443–450.

Watanabe, Y., Matsushita, T., Bhandari, M., Zdero, R., & Schemitsch, E. H. (2010). Ultrasound for fracture healing: current evidence. *Journal of Orthopaedical Trauma, 24,* S56-S61.

Westendorf, J. J., Kahler, R. A., & Schroeder, T. M. (2004). Wnt signaling in osteoblasts and bone diseases. *Gene, 341,* 19–39.

Wrana, J. L., Maeno, M., Hawrylyshyn, B., Yao, K. L., Domenicucci, C., & Sodek, J. (1988). Differential effects of transforming growth factor-beta on the synthesis of extracellular matrix proteins by normal fetal rat calvarial bone cell populations. *Journal of Cell Biology, 106,* 915-924.

Wu, C.-C., Lewallen, D. G., Bolander, M. E., Bronk, J., Kinnick, R., & Greenleaf, J. F. (1996). Exposure to low intensity ultrasound stimulates aggrecan gene expression by cultured chondrocytes. *Transactions of the Orthopaedic Research Society, 21,* 590.

Yang, K. H., Parvizi, J., Wang, S. J., Lewallen, D. G., Kinnick, R. R., Greenleaf, J. F., & Bolander, M. E. (1996). Exposure to low-intensity ultrasound increases aggrecan gene expression in a rat femur fracture model. *Journal of Orthopaedic Research, 14,* 802-809.

Index

#

1,25-dihydroxyvitamin D3, 220, 221, 244
18β, 229
2D, 96, 137, 139, 179, 182, 198
3D, 9, 10, 49, 56, 100, 104, 179, 180, 181
β-glycerophosphate, 230, 231

A

absorption, 55, 64, 66, 91, 130, 138, 168, 185, 205, 207
acceleration, 201, 216, 233, 238, 239, 243, 244
accuracy, 145, 154, 155, 157, 159, 160, 161, 164, 165
acoustic impedance, 60, 65, 79, 102, 103, 107, 147, 189
acoustical waves, 20
acoustics, 19, 20, 68, 72, 73, 82, 86, 87, 90, 105, 109, 110, 114, 140
active element, 75, 79
adenosine 5'-triphosphate, 227, 228, 244
adenylate cyclase, 216, 247
adiabatic bulk modulus, 68
adiabatic compressibility, 70
aggrecan, 211, 214, 216, 232, 249
algorithm, 47, 48, 49, 199
alignment, 150, 152, 154

alkaline phosphatase, 222, 229, 235
A-mode, 56, 89, 94, 95, 96, 97, 98, 107, 146
amplitude, 57, 68, 69, 78, 93, 94, 95, 97, 138, 145, 146, 151, 171, 173, 184, 185, 187
angiogenesis, 15, 42, 43, 205, 208, 210, 216, 235, 236, 240, 242
angiopoietin, 43
angle of divergence, 63
angle of incidence, 65
angular frequency, 82, 116, 174
angulated fracture, 44
anisotropic, 12, 19, 25, 32, 103, 107, 113, 122, 123
anisotropy, 19, 25, 28, 30, 33, 35, 139, 179, 180
apodization, 56
apparent density, 31, 32, 33
apparent integrated backscatter, 106, 107
apposition rate, 6
area, 8, 19, 22, 23, 39, 97, 152, 189, 223, 232, 235, 240, 241, 247
arrays, 56
artifacts, 86
ascorbic acid, 230, 231
assays, 217
assessment, vii, ix, xiv, 38, 94, 101, 102, 108, 134, 136, 138, 139, 141, 143, 145, 146, 150, 152, 154, 155, 162, 167, 168,

169, 172, 173, 175, 177, 192, 197, 199, 232, 233, 238
asymmetric, 132
atoms, 20, 114
ATP, 227, 228
attenuation, 55, 56, 66, 67, 91, 94, 96, 105, 106, 108, 125, 130, 140, 167, 168, 171, 175, 184, 185, 186, 198, 200, 201
attenuation coefficient, 66, 67, 130
autologous bone graft, 189
availability, 158
axial resolution, 99, 100, 109
axial transmission, 11, 16, 134, 136, 137, 139, 140, 141, 167, 169, 170, 171, 173, 174, 175, 176, 179, 180, 181, 184, 187, 192, 193, 194, 195, 196, 197, 198, 200

B

backing, 75, 79, 80
backscatter coefficient, 89, 92, 105, 110, 140
backscattered, xiii, 90, 93, 104, 109, 130, 167, 168, 172, 200, 201
backscattering coefficient, 113, 130, 167, 168, 172
baffle, 83, 85
bandwidth, 61
battlefields, 158
beam axis, 63, 242
beam divergence, 66
beam width, 80
beamforming, xiv, 75, 81, 86
bedside ultrasound (BUS), 154, 157, 159, 163
bending, 21, 22, 46, 114, 177, 234
bending testing, 177
bidirectional, 174
biocompatibility, 239
bioeffects, viii, 197, 205, 206
biomechanics, xiv, 20, 34, 35, 39, 48, 50, 51, 138, 140, 177, 198, 200
biopsies, 240
biot, 113, 114, 125, 126, 128, 139, 140, 141
blind, 155, 240, 245, 247

block diagram, 95, 96, 97, 98
blood flow, 89, 101, 102, 214, 238
blood red cells, 101
blood supply, 13, 42, 45
B-mode, 56, 89, 96, 97, 98, 100, 102, 107, 145, 146, 147, 148, 149, 150, 152, 153, 154, 155, 157, 158, 159, 160
bone growth, 12, 13, 14, 15, 40, 208, 209, 211, 216, 218, 220, 221, 222, 225, 226, 243, 244, 245, 249
bone healing, ix, xiii, xiv, xv, 13, 16, 34, 37, 38, 39, 40, 41, 42, 43, 46, 47, 48, 49, 50, 51, 56, 90, 113, 131, 132, 133, 138, 140, 146, 154, 167, 168, 169, 174, 175, 176, 177, 178, 179, 180, 181, 182, 183, 185, 186, 188, 189, 192, 193, 194, 195, 196, 197, 198, 199, 200, 201, 202, 205, 208, 210, 211, 212, 213, 214, 215, 216, 219, 220, 227, 231, 232, 233, 234, 235, 236, 238, 239, 240, 241, 242, 243, 244, 245, 246, 247, 248, 249
bone lining cells, 3, 5, 6, 7, 8
bone mineral density (BMD), 10, 108, 177, 232, 233, 234, 239, 241, 248
bone morphogenetic proteins (BMP), 37, 42, 226, 247
bone regeneration, 13, 14, 16, 37, 40, 41, 42, 43, 45, 46, 47, 49, 50, 151, 179, 197, 205, 206, 208, 210, 212, 216, 238, 241
bone strength, ix, xv, 19, 20, 21, 22, 31, 33, 41, 82, 114, 168, 169, 199, 200, 231, 233, 234, 243, 248
bone volume fraction, 9, 10, 31, 238
bone-mimicking, 176
bony collar, 223
bony matrix volume, 31
born approximation, 130
boundaries, 64, 83, 91, 96, 97, 100
bovine, 26, 30, 35, 139, 174, 184, 185, 186, 187, 194, 195, 198
bridging, 46, 188, 235, 236, 237, 238
bubbles, 205, 208
bulk modulus, 24, 47, 126
burst, 96, 220, 231

Index

C

calcein, 229
calcification zone, 15
calcified cartilage, 13
calcitonin, 8
calcium, 4, 5, 147, 150, 195, 196, 205, 209, 210, 212, 214, 216, 220, 246
callus, xiv, 37, 38, 39, 40, 41, 46, 47, 49, 109, 146, 152, 154, 163, 167, 177, 179, 180, 183, 185, 187, 188, 189, 190, 191, 192, 193, 197, 199, 206, 211, 216, 232, 234, 235, 236, 237, 239, 241, 242, 243, 248
cancellous bone, 4, 10, 27, 128, 131, 139, 140, 141, 198, 199, 200
cancer, 163, 205, 209, 212
cardiology, 56, 94
cartilage, 3, 12, 13, 14, 15, 38, 43, 44, 45, 47, 48, 188, 193, 205, 210, 211, 212, 216, 223, 232, 235, 236
catalysis, 207
cathode ray tube, 95
cavitation, 205, 208, 209, 211
cell culture, 227
cell population, 224, 225, 249
center frequency, 60
ceramic, 75, 77
c-fos, 211, 221, 222
chelant, 195
chemotactic, 43, 49
chirps, 100
chondroblasts, 14, 41
chondrocytes, 13, 14, 15, 42, 47, 214, 216, 220, 233, 246, 249
Christoffel, 113, 122, 123, 124
clear zone, 8
coagulation, 207, 209
coaxial cable, 75, 79, 80
cohort, 155
collagen, 4, 5, 6, 7, 10, 12, 14, 27, 32, 44, 108, 208, 217, 218, 226, 238, 245
combat theater, 158, 162, 164
comminuted fractures, 158
compact bone, 5, 9, 10, 12, 34
complex source strength, 82
compliance, 22, 26, 27
complications, 38, 239, 241
compression, 21, 22, 28, 33, 44, 45, 46, 56, 57, 58, 59, 69, 77, 100, 114, 117
computerized tomography, 177
concavity, 80
condensation, 68
conduction, 205, 207
configuration, 84, 85, 102, 179, 180, 184, 196
connective tissue, 38, 44, 47
connector, 79
consolidation, 176, 179, 189, 191, 241
constant equilibrium density, 82
constructive interference, 62, 78, 79
continuity, 34, 37, 38, 154
continuous wave, 80
contrast-media imaging, 100
control, 14, 108, 109, 110, 139, 140, 155, 168, 175, 198, 199, 200, 201, 202, 217, 221, 222, 223, 224, 230, 231, 232, 233, 234, 235, 236, 237, 238, 239, 240, 241
correlations, 50, 175, 177
cortical bone, 10, 11, 15, 16, 20, 26, 27, 28, 32, 33, 34, 35, 41, 48, 103, 113, 131, 138, 141, 146, 147, 177, 179, 180, 183, 184, 185, 186, 191, 194, 195, 196, 198, 200, 201, 233, 237
cortical interruption, 155
corticotomy, 154
COX-2, 219, 220, 222
CP-Ti implants, 238
critical angle, 133, 135, 235
cross product, 21
CRT, 95, 96
crystal lattice, 55, 58, 59
Curie, 76, 87
curvature radius, 80, 81
cutting cones, 38, 46
cyclic tissue loading, 45
cylindrical waves, 70
cytokines, 8, 40, 43, 218, 247
cytoskeletal filaments, 209

D

daily activities, 240
daily-changing healing models, 192
damping, 114
default, 38
deformations, 20, 21
deformities, 154
delayed union, 38, 41, 42, 192, 212, 238, 239, 240, 245, 247
demodulator, 96
density, 3, 8, 9, 10, 31, 32, 35, 60, 68, 69, 115, 120, 130, 172, 214, 232, 233, 234, 238, 248
depth, 66, 67, 96, 127, 154
dermatology, 102
destructive interference, 62, 130
detrimental effect, 207
deviatoric strain, 47
diabetes mellitus, 232
diagnosis, x, xiv, 90, 93, 94, 145, 154, 155, 157, 158, 160, 161, 162, 163, 164, 165, 239
diaphysis, 5, 15, 171, 223
dielectric constant, 77
differentiation, 3, 6, 13, 37, 40, 42, 43, 44, 45, 47, 213, 220, 229, 230, 231, 242, 245
differentiation factors, 40
diffraction, 80, 104, 105, 109, 184
diffusion, 209
discontinuity, 145, 155, 158, 161, 210, 211
discrimination, 108, 168, 177
dispersion, 117, 119, 131, 132, 179, 198
displacement, 23, 96, 120, 152, 154
display, 95, 97
disruption, 38, 209
distortional stress, 37, 44
distraction osteogenesis, 154, 163, 215, 232, 233, 238, 240, 242, 243, 248
disturbance, 55, 56, 57, 59, 206
DNA, 209, 218
doppler, 56, 89, 101, 102, 109, 238
double-blind, 239, 240, 245
drilled holes, 216
drug, 209, 233

dual-energy X-ray absorptiometry, 239
Dussik brothers, 56, 168
dynamic focusing, 56

E

echo, 89, 94, 95, 97, 99, 109, 146, 167
echogenic line, 96
EDTA, 195
effectiveness, 155
efflux, 216, 242
elastic cartilage, 14
elastic constants, 25, 26, 123, 126
elastic restoring forces, 115
elasticity, 14, 24, 38, 102, 114
elderly, 212, 239
electric field, 76, 77
ELISA, 218
embryonic, 3, 12, 13
emergency rooms, 38, 108, 157
emitter, 81, 83, 128, 167, 169, 173, 184
endochondral ossification, 3, 12, 13, 14, 37, 38, 39, 40, 41, 43, 46, 47, 146, 212, 223, 233, 235, 236, 246
endothelial cells, 43, 220, 221, 244
enhancement, 13, 16, 40, 50, 51, 177, 178, 197, 200, 205, 210, 212, 213, 216, 232, 236, 237, 241, 242, 244
enzymes, 7, 205, 207, 210, 211, 216
epiphyseal plate, 3, 14, 15
epiphysis, 9, 15, 33, 156, 161, 164
equation of continuity, 55, 68, 69
equation of motion, 55, 68, 69, 119
equation of state, 55, 68
equilibrium, 20, 68, 115
equilibrium position, 20
erythrocytes, 101
evidences, xiii, xiv, 49, 138, 146, 154, 160, 162, 169, 175, 197, 212, 215, 216, 234, 238, 241
ex vivo, 108, 179
exam, 102, 150, 207
excess pressure, 57, 58, 60, 68
exogen, 216, 244

Index

experimental, x, 49, 127, 138, 141, 171, 176, 185, 186, 187, 188, 194, 195, 196, 197, 198, 199, 200, 233, 237
experiments, x, 44, 130, 167, 179, 187, 217
extensibility, 208
external fixation index, 240
external fixation time, 240
extracellular matrix, 14, 38, 42, 43, 47, 209, 232, 249

F

failure, 22, 175, 190, 232, 238
failure point, 22
false-positive, 161, 162
far field, 55, 63, 64, 80, 84, 85
Faran cylinder model, 113, 130
FEA, 37, 46, 47
femur, 10, 16, 27, 28, 108, 149, 151, 158, 169, 186, 187, 194, 195, 198, 216, 231, 249
fibroblast growth factor (FGF), 42, 218, 247
fibrocartilage, 14, 39, 44, 45, 46
fibrous matrix, 45
first arriving signal (FAS), 167, 173, 174, 179, 180, 182, 185, 186, 192
flat bones, 5
flexibility, 3, 5
flexural, 132, 248
fluid velocity, 47
focal width, 80
focusing, xiii, xiv, 62, 75, 80, 81, 86, 96
follow-up, xiv, 155, 157, 162
force, 19, 20, 23, 25, 76, 115, 189
fourier transform, 55, 61, 92, 174
fracture, ix, x, xiii, xiv, xv, 13, 14, 16, 19, 22, 27, 34, 37, 38, 39, 40, 41, 42, 43, 45, 46, 47, 48, 49, 50, 51, 56, 94, 108, 113, 131, 133, 138, 145, 146, 150, 152, 153, 154, 155, 156, 157, 158, 159, 160, 161, 162, 163, 164, 167, 168, 169, 173, 174, 175, 176, 177, 178, 179, 180, 184, 185, 187, 188, 189, 192, 193, 194, 195, 196, 197, 198, 199, 200, 201, 205, 206, 208, 210, 211, 212, 213, 214, 215, 216, 219, 220, 227, 228, 231, 232, 233, 234, 235, 236, 237, 238, 239, 240, 241, 242, 243, 244, 245, 247, 248, 249
fracture healing, ix, xiii, xiv, xv, 13, 16, 34, 37, 38, 39, 40, 41, 42, 43, 46, 47, 48, 49, 50, 51, 56, 113, 131, 133, 138, 146, 154, 167, 168, 169, 174, 175, 176, 177, 178, 179, 180, 187, 188, 189, 192, 193, 194, 195, 196, 197, 199, 200, 201, 205, 208, 210, 211, 212, 213, 214, 215, 216, 219, 220, 227, 231, 232, 233, 234, 235, 236, 238, 239, 240, 241, 242, 243, 244, 247, 248, 249
fracture resistance, 27, 189
Fraunhofer zone, 55, 63, 64
frequency, 9, 17, 55, 56, 60, 61, 62, 66, 67, 78, 81, 82, 89, 92, 94, 100, 101, 103, 105, 107, 108, 109, 110, 113, 125, 126, 128, 129, 131, 132, 138, 139, 140, 158, 168, 171, 172, 174, 179, 184, 189, 197, 198, 199, 200, 201, 202, 206, 218, 220, 221, 223, 226, 227, 231, 232
frequency spectrum, 61, 67
fresh, 215, 238, 239, 241, 245, 248
Fresnel zone, 55, 63, 64
Friedrich Pauwels, 44

G

gap, 42, 46, 47, 48, 49, 51, 152, 154, 168, 176, 177, 179, 184, 185, 187, 188, 190, 192, 193, 194, 195, 196, 197, 211, 229, 236, 241, 246, 247
gap junction inhibitor, 229
gas, 56, 94, 100, 205, 208
gastroenterology, 94
gene, 205, 209, 210, 211, 212, 216, 226, 232, 235, 245, 247, 249
gene transfection, 205, 209
geometry, 49, 104, 179, 180, 185
glass, 114
granular, 89, 100, 147
gray-scale, 96, 97, 146, 163
growth factors, 42, 43, 222
growth plate, 14, 15

Index

guidance, xv, 155, 159, 162
guided waves, 113, 114, 131, 132, 140, 173, 179, 180, 183
guinea pigs, 175
gynecology, 56, 94, 201

H

harmonic imaging, 100, 110
harmonic wave, 70
harmonics, 79, 100
Haversian systems, 4, 12
health care, 38
heart chambers, 89, 102
heating, 206, 207
hematopoiesis, 4
hematopoietic tissue, 13
hemocallotasis, 239
hemorrhage, 209
hemostasis, 205, 209
heterogeneous, 89, 90, 91, 113, 114, 175
high-resolution, 9, 10, 110, 151
high-resolution synchrotron radiation, 9, 10
Hilbert transform, 97
histology, vii, 3, 5, 15, 231, 234
hollow pipes, 113, 131
homogeneous, 68, 90, 91, 114, 131, 138, 197
Hooke's law, 25
hormones, 8, 40
horses, 234, 246
human trials, 216
Huygen's principle, 55, 62, 63, 81
hyaline cartilage, 3, 12, 13, 14, 15, 44
hydrophones, 63, 64
hydrostatic pressure, 44, 45
hydrostatic stress, 37, 44, 45
hydroxyapatite, 5
hyperthermia, 209, 214
hypertrophic zone, 14, 15
hypertrophy, 13

I

IBC, 93
IL, 43, 218, 226, 247
images, 56, 89, 93, 96, 100, 102, 103, 106, 108, 109, 110, 146, 147, 148, 149, 150, 152, 153, 154, 155, 157, 158, 159, 160, 161, 162, 168, 189
imaging modes, 56
immobilization, 41, 46
immune response, 205, 209
immunization, 209
immunohistochemical staining, 232
implantation, 177
implants, 46, 237, 238, 244
in vitro, x, xiii, 10, 16, 110, 146, 168, 169, 175, 179, 184, 185, 186, 187, 194, 198, 200, 208, 212, 213, 216, 217, 220, 223, 233, 237, 238, 241, 242, 244, 246, 247
in vivo, 44, 47, 48, 50, 108, 140, 146, 168, 169, 175, 179, 200, 208, 212, 233, 237, 238, 242, 244, 246
incident intensity, 65, 92
induction, 38, 205, 210, 211, 215, 219, 220, 223, 245
infections, 38
inflammatory phase, 40
inhibitor, 219, 220
inhomogeneous, 90, 91, 113, 125
initial connective tissue, 180
injury, 40, 42, 50, 51, 148, 149, 150, 155, 157, 161, 164, 165, 176, 208, 210, 211, 214, 245, 248
instantaneous pressure, 68
insulin like growth factor (IGF), 43, 211, 222
intensity, 51, 63, 64, 65, 66, 67, 82, 83, 91, 92, 145, 151, 177, 178, 200, 206, 207, 208, 209, 213, 214, 216, 219, 220, 222, 225, 226, 227, 229, 230, 231, 232, 233, 234, 235, 236, 237, 242, 243, 244, 245, 246, 247, 248, 249
interfaces, 27, 51, 64, 146, 147
interference, 62, 78, 81, 91, 184
interfragmentary movements, 46

Index

interleukin, 43, 218
intermediate stiffness callus, 180
internal fixation, 155, 176
internal medicine, 94
interrater reliability, 157
intramembranous ossification, 12, 13, 232
intraoperative, 155
intravascular imaging, 102
inverse piezoelectric effect, 76
ion, 205, 209, 216
ion channels, 205, 209
ionizing, 89, 93, 151, 197
irregular bones, 5
irregularity, 145, 155
isotropic, 25, 26, 29, 68, 113, 122, 123, 125, 131, 180

J

joints, 12, 14, 94, 156, 208

L

lacunae, 6, 7, 8, 14
lamb, 131, 132, 138, 179, 197
Lamé constants, 71
lamellae, 4, 10, 11, 12
lamellar bone, 12, 32
lateral resolution, 99, 102
lateral wave, 133, 134, 135, 136, 137, 138, 179, 184, 185, 197
lead zirconate titanate, 75, 77
leakage, 183
linearized continuity equation, 69
linearized wave equation, 55, 69
LiUS, 177, 178
load, 19, 21, 22, 24, 33, 49, 175, 233
load-deformation, 21, 24, 33
long bones, 3, 5, 9, 10, 14, 15, 27, 33, 131, 132, 140, 154, 156, 171, 176, 177, 179, 180, 181, 199, 200, 201
longitudinal strain, 24
longitudinal wave, 58, 119, 125, 137
low-cost, 89, 145, 158, 197

low-intensity pulsed ultrasound (LIPUS), x, xiv, 197, 205, 210, 211, 212, 213, 214, 215, 216, 219, 220, 223, 226, 227, 229, 230, 231, 232, 233, 234, 235, 236, 237, 238, 239, 240, 241, 242, 243, 245, 246, 247, 248

M

magnetic resonance, 106
management, x, 46, 155, 212
manipulation, 77, 155, 156
maps, 190
marrow, 3, 4, 7, 9, 13, 15, 31, 33, 48, 113, 128, 129, 131, 182, 221, 222, 226, 229, 242, 246, 247, 248
masses, 55, 58, 59
matching layer, 75, 79, 80
maturation, 15, 205, 210, 216, 248
mean scatterer spacing (MSS), 167, 168, 172, 202
mechanical effects, 205, 208, 217
mechanical equilibrium, 21
mechanics, vii, 3, 5, 16, 19, 20, 34, 35, 51, 105, 139
mechanobiology, 16, 37, 43, 44, 45, 50
mechanotransduction, 209
medicine, 5, 50, 56, 60, 75, 94, 95, 101, 107, 108, 109, 110, 111, 132, 140, 141, 152, 153, 156, 163, 164, 168, 179, 186, 187, 189, 190, 191, 192, 193, 198, 199, 200, 201, 206, 213, 214, 217, 221, 225, 228, 234, 235, 236, 237, 242, 243, 244, 245, 246, 247, 248
membrane, 8, 189, 205, 208, 209, 210
mesenchymal cells, 3, 6, 12, 13, 40, 42, 43, 44, 47, 242
meta-analysis, 200, 213, 215, 238, 248
metabolism, 5, 90, 219, 242, 246
metal case, 79
metal plates, 46
metalloproteinases, 43
metaphysis, 238
microarchitecture, 9
microdamage, 32

microscope, 102
microstreaming, 205, 208
midshaft, 156, 233
military forces, 158, 162
mineral apposition rate, 233, 240, 247
mineralization, 3, 5, 6, 10, 12, 13, 16, 31, 192, 194, 195, 196, 197, 200, 229, 236, 241
mismatch, 129, 147, 185, 207, 210, 211
mitogen-activated protein kinase (MAPK), 229
MLO-Y4, 230, 231
modeling, x, 46, 49, 50, 130, 140, 180, 181, 199, 201
models, 11, 16, 37, 46, 47, 49, 87, 113, 114, 129, 130, 140, 146, 175, 179, 182, 183, 185, 188, 192, 193, 197, 198, 202, 213, 215, 216, 231, 241
modulus of elasticity, 24, 34, 175, 232
molecular signaling, 37, 38
moment equilibrium, 20
monitoring, xiii, 133, 146, 167, 168, 174, 175, 176, 177, 178, 179, 180, 194, 195, 196, 197, 200, 201, 239
monocytes, 7, 8, 42, 43, 217, 218, 243
motion, 55, 56, 62, 69, 91, 101, 125, 132, 152, 184
mRNA, 216, 219, 220, 222, 245
multi-array, 96
multi-centre, 240, 245
multivariate regression, 189
muscle, xiii, 4, 5, 27, 49, 64, 93, 146, 147, 148, 150, 210, 214
muscle insertion, 27

N

nanoparticles, 209
near field, 55, 63, 64, 80, 242
necrosis, 14, 43, 209, 218
neonatal care, 145, 151, 162
network, 10, 107, 192
neutrophils, 212
Newton, 20, 69
nitric oxide, 223, 241, 247

non-destructive testing (NDT), 113, 131
nonrigid fixation, 46
non-specular reflection, 55, 64, 65
nonsteroidal anti-inflammatory drugs (NSAID), 233, 245
nonthermal effects, 205, 206, 208
nonunion, 38, 193, 232, 240, 245, 248
normal mode expansion, 180
novice, 155, 157
numerical modeling, 46
nurses, 158, 159, 160, 164

O

oblique, 158, 185, 186, 187, 198
obstetrics, 56, 94, 201
occult fractures, 155, 164
ophthalmology, 102, 110
organ, 91
orthopedics, 56, 94, 164, 247, 248
orthotropic, 25, 26, 28, 29, 35
oscilloscope, 95, 128
osseointegration, 237, 238, 244
ossification, 3, 12, 13, 14, 15, 41, 47, 180, 197
ossified callus, 180
osteoblasts, 3, 5, 6, 7, 8, 12, 13, 41, 42, 43, 47, 217, 218, 219, 220, 221, 223, 224, 225, 226, 227, 228, 230, 241, 242, 243, 244, 245, 247, 249
osteocalcin, 5, 211, 222, 235
osteoclasts, 3, 5, 6, 7, 8, 232
osteocytes, 3, 5, 6, 7, 8, 12, 230, 231, 245
osteogenesis, 212, 216, 226, 232, 238, 240
osteoid, 6, 7, 12, 240, 247
osteomalacia, 38
osteons, 4, 12, 27, 28, 34
osteoporosis, 38, 108, 131, 168, 197
osteoprogenitor cells, 7, 43
osteoprotegerin, 227
osteotomy, 178, 189, 190, 191, 200, 201, 216, 231, 233, 234, 244, 246, 248
oxygen radicals, 212, 214
oxygen tension, 45, 214

P

Paget's disease, 38
pain, xiii, 40, 208, 240
Palacos, 186
Paley index, 241
palpation, 155
parametric ultrasound imaging, 89, 106
parathormone, 8
particle displacement, 57, 58, 114, 117
particle displacement field, 114
particle velocity, 57, 58, 60, 69, 119, 120, 125
particles, 20, 23, 55, 57, 58, 66
pathological fractures, 38
pathways, 209, 210, 211, 227
PDLLA membranes, 189
peak load, 232
penetration, 130, 154
perfusion, 205, 207
perichondrium, 13
period, ix, xiii, 32, 56, 57, 60, 95, 173, 190, 206, 233, 241
periosteum, 12, 13, 15
permeability, 46, 125, 139, 205, 208, 209
PGE2, 219, 220, 223, 224, 225, 230, 231, 245
phantom, 110, 176
phase, 40, 41, 47, 62, 69, 78, 79, 83, 117, 119, 125, 127, 128, 131, 154, 171, 175, 212, 214
phase speed, 69
phosphate, 4, 5, 222
phosphorylation, 229
physical therapists, xiii, 206
physician, 157
physis, 14
piezoelectric effect, xiv, 76, 77
piezoelectric strain coefficient, 76
piezoelectrically stiffened constant, 77
piezoelectricity, 75, 76, 77, 86, 87
piston, 75, 85
placebo, 240, 245
plane waves, 63, 92, 113, 122
plaster casts, 46
plastic deformation, 19, 22
plasticity, 114
plate waves, 131
platelet-derived growth factor (PDGF), 43, 220, 221
plywood-like arrangement, 10
point-of-care, 155, 157, 165
Poisson ratio, 19, 24
poling, 75, 77
pore, 47, 125, 127
poroelastic material, 46
poromechanical model, 113
porosity, 3, 9, 11, 16, 27, 31, 34, 47, 103, 125, 126, 189
portability, 145, 158
potassium, 216, 242
power radiated, 82, 83
predictions, 192
pressure amplitude, 82, 84
pressure field, 82, 83, 84, 85
primary bone, 12
primary fracture healing, 38, 46
probe, 75, 79, 80, 86, 97, 146, 174, 194, 196, 207
proliferation, 3, 13, 43, 49, 209, 217, 220, 227, 228, 230, 231, 232, 238, 243, 245
proliferative zone, 15
proportional limit, 19, 22
prospective, 155, 239, 240, 243, 245
prostaglandin, 219, 220, 223, 224, 225, 245, 247
proteoglycans, 5, 14
pseudoarthrosis, 38, 41, 44, 151
pulse inversion imaging, 100
pulse length, 61, 99
pulse repetition frequency, 95
pulsed operation, 80
pulse-echo, 102, 103, 167, 169, 170, 172
PZT, 75, 77, 233

Q

qPCR, 234
quantitative real-time polymerase chain reaction, 234

quantitative ultrasound (QUS), x, xiii, xiv, 10, 16, 38, 56, 92, 95, 105, 108, 133, 167, 168, 169, 171, 172, 173, 175, 176, 177, 189, 192, 197, 199, 200
quasi-periodic, 172, 201

R

rabbit, 175, 233, 238, 247, 248
radar, 56
radiofrequency signal, 95
radiograph, 150, 152, 153, 154, 159, 178
radius, 16, 62, 63, 80, 81, 82, 91, 92, 93, 103, 127, 140, 152, 153, 154, 155, 156, 157, 163, 169, 216, 243
randomized, 197, 212, 215, 234, 239, 240, 243, 245, 247
RANKL, 227
rarefaction, 56, 58, 69
rat, 151, 214, 215, 226, 229, 232, 233, 234, 236, 238, 242, 246, 247, 248, 249
Rayleigh-Lamb, 131
real-time, 89, 93, 96, 159, 162
receiver, 75, 77, 104, 134, 135, 167, 169, 173, 176, 179, 184, 192
recruitment, 3, 13
reduction, 19, 42, 95, 109, 152, 153, 154, 155, 156, 159, 162, 163, 212, 237, 240
reference, x, 93, 169, 170, 171, 173
reflection, 64, 65, 66, 78, 93, 104, 107
reflection coefficient, 93
reflector, 89, 93, 94, 95, 96, 103, 167, 169
refraction, 55, 64, 65, 66
regeneration, 14, 16, 37, 41, 43, 45, 46, 49, 50, 152, 179, 205, 208, 210
region of interest, 93
regression, 172, 192, 193
rehabilitation, 206, 213, 248
reliability, 162
relief, xiii, 208
remodeling, 8, 11, 12, 27, 37, 38, 40, 41, 43, 146, 188, 208, 234, 235, 236, 237, 242
remodeling phase, 37, 40, 41
reparation, 40
reparative phase, 40, 41

repetition frequency, 221, 231
resistance, 114
resolution, 91, 94, 99, 100, 109, 151, 161, 189, 190, 199
resonance, 78
resting zone, 15
retrospective, 155
Reuss bulk modulus, 29, 30
Reuss shear modulus, 29
RF signals, 98
rigid fixation, 46
rigidity, 22, 41, 113
risk, ix, x, 169
ROI, 93
ruffled border, 8
Runx2, 226, 235

S

sample, 93, 102, 104, 105, 107, 127, 128, 129, 157, 167, 169, 171, 172, 173, 175, 194, 195, 239, 240
SATA, 215, 216, 217, 218, 220, 223, 226, 231, 232, 233, 234, 238
SATP, 224, 226
sawbones, 184, 186
scanning, 34, 89, 96, 97, 102, 103, 109, 161, 189, 195, 196, 199
scanning acoustic microscopy (SAM), 34, 89, 102, 103, 189, 190, 195, 196, 197
scar, 208
scattered power, 92
scatterer, 89, 91, 92, 94, 95, 99, 101, 201
scattering, vii, xiv, 55, 65, 66, 89, 90, 91, 92, 107, 109, 110, 111, 125, 129, 130, 138, 139, 140, 146, 172, 184, 199
scattering cross-section, 92
screws, 46, 242, 244
secondary bone, 12
self-heating, 207
semi-rigid, 189
sensitivity, 145, 154, 155, 158, 159, 161, 162, 180, 194, 199, 240
sesamoid bones, 5
setup, 127, 128, 171, 176, 181

shadowing, 96, 97, 108, 147, 148, 149, 154
shaft, 5, 10, 131, 156, 157, 231, 240
sham, 224, 225, 226, 229, 237, 239, 241, 247
shear, 19, 21, 22, 23, 24, 25, 26, 28, 29, 30, 102, 114, 116, 117, 119, 126, 131, 132
shear elastic anisotropy, 28
shear modulus, 24, 25, 28, 126
shear stress, 23
sheep, 39, 177, 178, 179, 189, 190, 191, 200, 201, 215, 233, 244
shell, 10, 27, 100, 131, 167, 171
shielding, 79
shift, 89, 101, 232
short bones, 5
short-time Fourier transform, 92
sialoprotein, 222
side lobes, 85, 86
signaling molecules, 8, 37, 40, 42, 208, 209
simple source, 82, 83
simsonic, 192
simulation, 50, 134, 137, 139, 158, 159, 177, 181, 185, 188, 194, 195, 196, 198, 199, 200
single-element, 79, 80, 96
singular value decomposition, 175, 202
skin, 64, 102, 109, 127, 146, 147, 209, 242
slice, 194, 195, 196
slow wave, 125
snapshots, 183, 185, 188
Snell's law, 66
soft callus, 180, 210
soft tissue, ix, 4, 9, 31, 32, 42, 45, 60, 89, 93, 94, 106, 107, 108, 131, 140, 146, 147, 150, 151, 162, 176, 179, 183, 205, 208, 212
software, 182, 183
solid mechanics, 19, 20, 34, 114
sonar, 56
sonographers, 155
sonopermeabilization, 209, 213
sonotransfection, 209, 213
sound pressure level (SPL), 167, 173, 184, 186, 187, 192

source, 43, 55, 56, 57, 62, 78, 82, 83, 84, 85, 86, 101, 134, 135, 137, 192, 207, 208
spasm, 208
specificity, 145, 154, 158, 159, 161, 162, 240
speckle, 89, 91, 100, 109, 147
specular reflection, 64, 65
speed, 56, 57, 60, 66, 78, 82, 85, 99, 105, 106, 108, 167, 168, 171, 197, 202
speed amplitude, 82, 85
speed of sound (SOS), 60, 66, 78, 82, 105, 106, 108, 167, 168, 169, 171, 175, 176, 197
spherical wave, 55, 62, 63, 133, 134
springs, 55, 58, 59
SR-PLLA, 239
stage, 41, 179, 180, 181, 183, 188
stainless-steel pin, 233
stasis, 208
stationary waves, 208
stiff callus, 180
stiffness, 3, 5, 22, 25, 27, 47, 48, 115, 119, 121, 122, 175, 190, 231, 232
stiffness tensor, 25
stimulation, x, xiii, xiv, 34, 38, 42, 47, 205, 206, 207, 208, 209, 210, 211, 212, 213, 215, 216, 217, 219, 221, 223, 224, 225, 226, 227, 228, 229, 231, 232, 233, 234, 237, 238, 242, 243, 244, 245, 247, 248
strain, 19, 22, 23, 24, 25, 28, 33, 37, 39, 44, 45, 46, 47, 50, 76, 77, 114, 115, 116, 117, 120, 125
strain field, 114, 116, 117
streaming, 205, 208
strength, xv, 19, 20, 21, 22, 33, 41, 114, 168, 231, 233, 234, 243, 248
stress, 6, 19, 22, 23, 24, 25, 28, 32, 33, 37, 39, 44, 45, 46, 47, 50, 75, 76, 77, 114, 115, 116, 118, 120, 122, 125, 233, 239, 245, 247
stress field, 118, 120
stress-displacement equation, 114
stromal cells, 221, 222, 226, 229, 241, 242, 248

262 Index

surgery, 46, 94, 161, 163, 178, 189, 201, 232, 234, 235, 236, 238, 243, 244, 245, 246, 248
swelling, 40
symmetric gradient operator, 114
symmetry, 26, 132
symptom, 239
systematic review, 161, 163, 213, 215, 216, 238, 248

T

target, 34, 101
targeted delivery, 209
technical elastic constants, 26
temperature, 20, 90, 205, 206, 207, 211, 217, 227, 242
tendon, 14, 146, 147, 148, 149, 150
tension, 21, 22, 28, 45, 114
texture, 89, 100, 108, 147, 150
thermal effects, 205, 206, 210
thickness, 10, 66, 78, 79, 80, 102, 127, 128, 131, 132, 137, 138, 139, 171, 175, 180, 184, 194, 198, 232, 240, 247
threshold, 22
through-transmission, 56, 167, 168, 169
thymocytes, 216, 242
tibia, 27, 28, 49, 50, 157, 168, 171, 179, 189, 199, 234, 238, 239, 240, 243, 247
time gain compensation, 95
time-of-flight (TOF), 94, 95, 137, 167, 169, 171, 173, 196
tissue characterization, 56, 60, 72, 93, 167, 171
tissue differentiation, 37, 44, 46, 47, 48, 50, 51
tomography, 104, 105, 107, 110, 145, 155, 161, 162, 164, 197, 232, 233, 234
torque, 231, 232, 238
torsion, 21, 22, 46, 114
torsional, 47, 132
tortuosity, 126, 127, 139
toxicity, 209
trabeculae, 4, 33, 107, 129, 130, 234, 235

trabecular bone, 5, 9, 10, 11, 15, 16, 17, 19, 27, 31, 33, 34, 35, 106, 107, 113, 125, 128, 129, 130, 138, 140, 172, 198, 199
training, 111, 155, 158, 159
transcutaneous, 209, 233
transducer, 55, 62, 63, 75, 78, 79, 80, 81, 86, 89, 93, 94, 95, 96, 97, 98, 101, 102, 103, 105, 146, 152, 158, 161, 163, 167, 169, 175, 176, 184, 189, 207, 233, 242
transforming growth factor (TGF), 37, 42, 216, 226, 241, 247, 249
transient expression, 221
translational equation of motion, 115
transmission coefficient, 128
transmission scattering operator, 128
transmitted intensity, 65
transmitter, 75, 78, 104, 134, 135, 167, 169, 173, 176, 179
transosseous low-intensity pulsed ultrasound, 177
transverse fracture, 46, 179, 184, 186
transverse strain, 24
transverse wave, 58, 59, 125
trauma, 158, 164, 198, 214, 243, 244, 246, 247, 249
triage, 159, 162
triclinic, 123, 124
tumors, 38, 56, 168
turnover, 13
Type I collagen, 6, 238

U

ultimate load, 22
ultrasonic computed tomography (UCT), 89, 104, 105
ultrasonographers, 157
ultrasonography, 93, 145, 150, 151, 154, 155, 158, 159, 160, 161, 162, 163, 164, 238
ultrasound beam, 55, 62, 63, 64, 72, 80, 81, 101, 152, 154, 206
ultrasound imaging, 89, 90, 91, 93, 94, 99, 108, 146, 151, 155, 158, 163
upregulation, 208, 210, 235

uptake, 209, 216
urology, 94

V

VAS, 240
vascular proliferation, 41
vascular-endothelial growth factor (VEGF), 43, 218, 247
vascularization, 41, 235, 242
vasculature, 209
vectors, 20
velocity potential, 69, 70
vessels, 10, 13, 14, 43, 64, 89, 94, 101, 146, 208
vibrational motion, 20, 55, 58
video amplifier, 96
viscoelastic material, 32
viscoelasticity, 114
Visual Analogue Pain Scores, 240
volume, 9, 10, 14, 24, 31, 114, 125, 127, 129, 130, 138, 151, 154, 168, 172, 207, 229, 233, 240, 244, 245, 247, 248

W

water bath, 169
Wave2000, 182, 183, 184, 186
wavefront, 55, 56, 57, 62, 70, 71, 82, 133, 134
waveguides, 131
wavelength, 57, 60, 66, 78, 80, 82, 116, 125, 129, 175, 180
wavelet, 62, 201
wavenumber, 70, 82, 91, 131, 174
wearable, 177, 201
weight-bearing, 175
wireless, 177
Wistar, 151, 216, 233, 243
Wnt/β-catenin, 227
Wolff, xv, 20
World War, 56
wound, 208
woven bone, 12, 32, 237, 238

X

x-ray, ix, x, 93, 150, 156, 168, 178, 232, 233

Y

yield point, 19, 22, 32
Young's modulus, 19, 24, 25, 31, 32, 33, 34, 35, 46, 60, 71, 187, 197